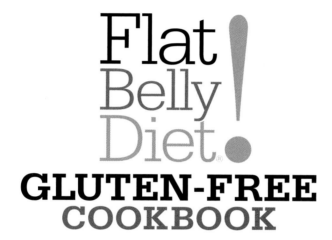

Flat Belly Diet!
GLUTEN-FREE COOKBOOK

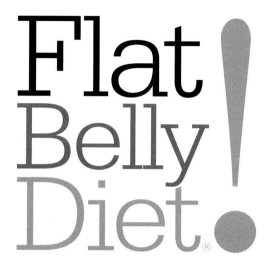

Flat Belly Diet!

GLUTEN-FREE
COOKBOOK

From the editors of **Prevention**®

RODALE®

This book is intended as a reference volume only, not as a medical manual. The information given here is designed to help you make informed decisions about your health. It is not intended as a substitute for any treatment that may have been prescribed by your doctor. If you suspect that you have a medical problem, we urge you to seek competent medical help.

Mention of specific companies, organizations, or authorities in this book does not imply endorsement by the author or publisher, nor does mention of specific companies, organizations, or authorities imply that they endorse this book, its author, or the publisher.

Internet addresses and telephone numbers given in this book were accurate at the time it went to press.

© 2013 by Rodale Inc.
Photographs © 2013 by Rodale Inc.

All rights reserved. No part of this publication may be reproduced or transmitted in any form or by any means, electronic or mechanical, including photocopying, recording, or any other information storage and retrieval system, without the written permission of the publisher.

Rodale books may be purchased for business or promotional use or for special sales. For information, please write to: Special Markets Department, Rodale Inc., 733 Third Avenue, New York, NY 10017

Prevention is a registered trademark of Rodale Inc.

Printed in the United States of America
Rodale Inc. makes every effort to use acid-free ♾, recycled paper ♻.

Photographs by Mitch Mandel/Rodale Images
Book design by Carol Angstadt

Library of Congress Cataloging-in-Publication Data is on file with the publisher.

ISBN 978-1-60961-940-4 hardcover

Distributed to the trade by Macmillan

2   4   6   8   10   9   7   5   3   1   hardcover

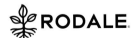

We inspire and enable people to improve their lives and the world around them.
For more of our products visit prevention.com.

For celiac sufferers and gluten-sensitive tummies everywhere—you're just meals away from a flatter belly.

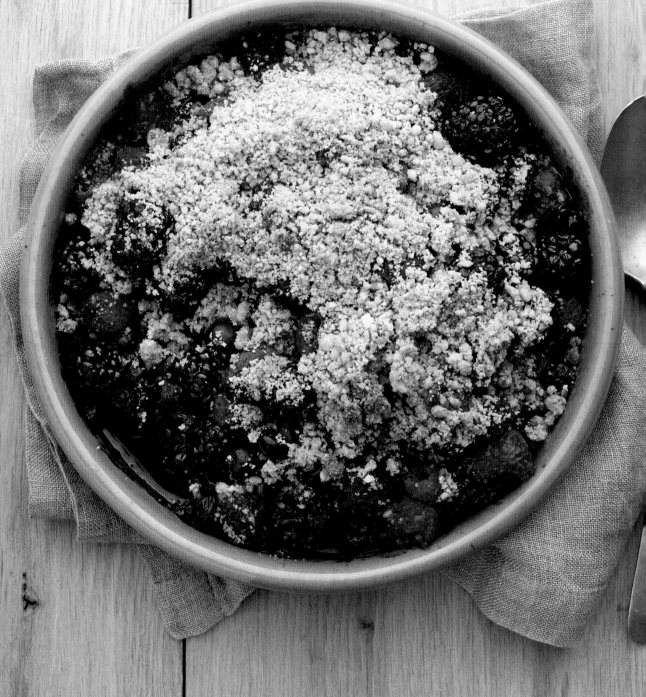

contents

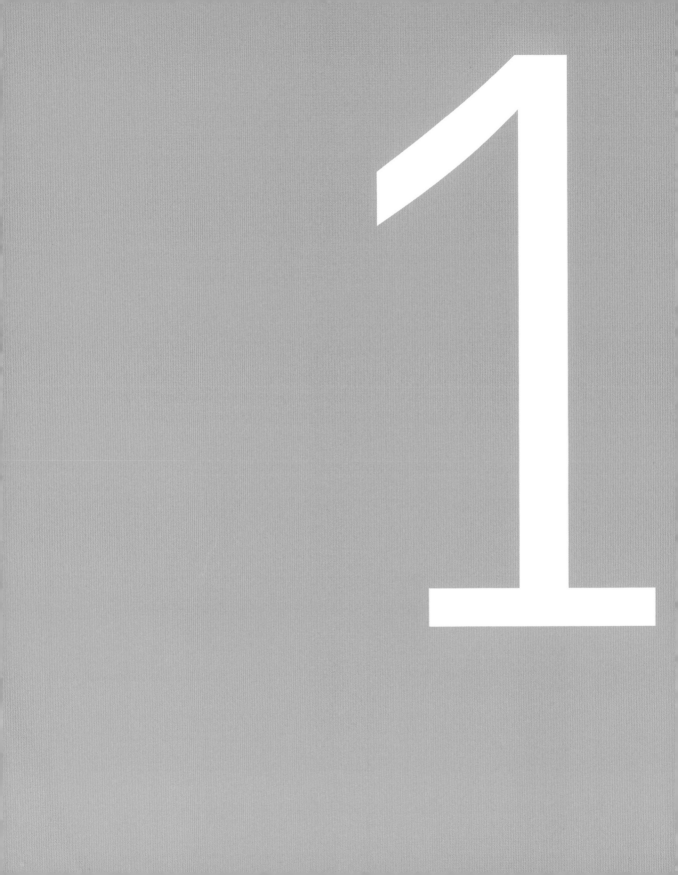

BREAK FREE FROM BELLY FAT!

Getting the flat belly you want by eating truly delicious foods may seem like a dream, but more than a million readers have used the proven program behind the original Flat Belly Diet to beat bloat and permanently go from flab to fab. Busy moms have slipped comfortably back into their skinny jeans; harried husbands have melted their guts into six-pack abs; and readers with diabetes have tamed their blood sugar and slimmed their sloping bellies. Now, it's your turn.

Trying to find a healthy eating plan that will help you shed pounds without causing pain and discomfort can be exceptionally difficult if you are sensitive to this one formidable foe. (Hint: It's an ingredient found in almost every processed food in the typical American diet.) Not sugar. Not even fat. No, you're up against *gluten*.

A protein found in wheat, barley, and rye, gluten is off-limits if you have celiac disease or if you have been diagnosed with, or suspect, a gluten sensitivity.

On the other hand, perhaps you are avoiding gluten by choice—someone in your family is sensitive, or maybe you know someone who feels better than ever on a gluten-free diet, and *wow*. You want in on their newfound energy, increased mental focus, and brighter mood—and who could blame you?

That's why we've modified our classic Flat Belly Diet to create a new regimen that literally gets at the core of your weight loss desires without a bit of gluten. No matter which camp you fall into, this belly-flattening eating plan takes gluten out of the picture while pumping up the flavor so that you can enjoy being on a diet that doesn't taste like one!

Whether you are a gluten-free veteran or starting this journey for the first time, the *Flat Belly Diet! Gluten-Free Cookbook* will help you reach your weight loss goals by combining our *New York Times* best-selling belly-shrinking formula with truly delicious gluten-free fare.

How does waking up to creamy Blueberry-Almond Breakfast Pudding (page 68) sound? (Drizzle on some maple syrup, too!) For lunch, enjoy savory Quinoa with Roasted Tomatoes, Walnuts, and Olives (page 135). For dinner, tuck into Chicken Cobbler with Cornmeal-Pepita Topping (page 186). Want dessert? Splurge on Dark Chocolate Mint Pudding (page 278) or jumbo Peanut Butter–Chocolate Chunk Cookies (page 271).

If these dishes sound too good to be true, take heart. They all share a powerful ingredient proven to punch out belly fat. The key is this: To shed belly fat, you've gotta eat fat—specifically, healthy fat—at every meal.

These healthy fats are *monounsaturated fatty acids*—MUFAs (pronounced moo-fahs), for short. We're talking the plant-based, ultrahealthy dietary fats found in some of the world's tastiest whole foods. There's compelling scientific evidence that MUFAs may target body fat where it's hardest to lose: in your belly. As a bonus, MUFAs promote satiety, that wonderful feeling of fullness that makes it easier to make healthy choices, brush off cravings, and whittle off belly inches.

The best part: Because MUFA-rich foods are some of the tastiest on the planet, you'll never feel deprived. (Hint: You get to eat chocolate.) Flat Belly Diet Gluten-Free is as flexible as it is delicious. You can follow our suggested menu or use our guidelines as inspiration to design your own. And as a look through the recipes will show, you can assemble a tasty meal, snack, or dessert in minutes.

Now, gluten-free aficionados, it's your turn to lose—deliciously. Follow the plan faithfully, and you *will* lose weight (especially in your belly), reignite your energy, and enhance your chances of living a longer, healthier life. But before we turn to the plan, let's set the record straight on fat—both the fat you eat and the fat you store.

Let's Start at the Beginning

This chapter is your Flat Belly Diet Gluten-Free crash course. You'll learn why MUFAs are unique among dietary fats, how they help fight chronic disease as well as obesity, and meet the five MUFA superstars that form the core of the diet. You'll also get the how-tos of eating the Flat Belly way, beginning with a 4-day Jumpstart and moving on to a 28-day eating plan that gives you flexibility, enables you to continue to shed pounds, and teaches you how to keep the weight off.

Once you're up to speed on the basic program, we'll spend Chapter 2 giving you more details on how you can do this plan *sans* gluten—and all the perks that come with it. You'll hear all about the research linking a gluten-free diet with a ton of fascinating health benefits, and you'll also learn to easily recognize and remove foods that contain gluten from your diet.

As you'll see, going gluten free doesn't mean giving up the pasta, pancakes, and sweets you love. If you need proof, now would be a good time to skim the recipes, which begin on page 68.

The Facts on Fat

Remember the ill-fated fat-free craze of the 1990s? Every supermarket aisle bulged with fat-free crackers, cookies, chips, ice cream . . . the list goes on. In fact, responding to America's concern about its fat intake, food manufacturers introduced more than 5,400 lower-fat foods between 1995 and 1997!

What triggered America's fat phobia? Here's a best guess from famed Harvard nutrition researcher Walter Willett, MD, in an article published in *Public Health Nutrition*. In the late 1980s, he writes, nutritionists stopped advising people to eat more heart-healthy polyunsaturated fat and less artery-clogging saturated fat. Instead, their recommendation was to eat less fat—period. It seems nutty now, but Dr. Willett theorizes that well-intentioned nutritionists may have doubted our ability to distinguish between different types of dietary fat. They were trying not to confuse us, and to recommend reducing our intake of fat across the board must have seemed like a good idea at the time.

Americans listened to the experts and did eat less fat. Yet—shockingly—bellies everywhere expanded. By the year 2000, a whopping 62 percent of adult Americans were overweight, up from 46 percent in 1980!

The "eat no fat" campaign may have contributed to the rise in obesity, Willett's article theorizes, because experts seemed to be saying that only calories from fat could make you fat. No wonder weight-conscious folks turned to carbohydrates! But we went waaay overboard on the carbs. This didn't help our hearts, either: Not surprisingly, even as medical technology improved during these years, the number of deaths from coronary heart disease in the United States began to plateau.

The high-protein diets that came along next were hardly any better. They gave the green light to all types of fat, even saturated fats (the kind that turn your arteries into sludgy tubes and raise the risk of heart disease). And while dieters did lose weight on these regimens, it quickly piled back on when the steak-and-eggs routine proved impossible to stick to in the long term.

Fortunately, some of the latest weight loss research has settled on a middle ground: Fat is a crucial component of a healthy diet—and a surprisingly vital piece of a successful weight loss plan. While you should opt for healthy fats more often than not, zapping all fat from your diet will leave you listless, cranky, and hungry. So please, if you still have a touch of fat phobia, lay it to rest and strive to strike a balance in your diet. This handy cheat sheet can help you reap the benefits of good fats and avoid the potential health risks of the bad.

THE BAD (SATURATED) FATS

Saturated fat is solid at room temperature, which is why it is also known as "solid fat." (Think butter or the thick marbling in a steak.) Found primarily in animal foods—milk, cheese, and meat—saturated fats raise levels of waxlike LDL ("bad") cholesterol in the blood. Excessive amounts can build up on artery walls and boost inflammation, restricting bloodflow and increasing the risk of cardiovascular disease and strokes. While animal products are the main source of saturated fats, tropical oils like coconut or palm (or palm kernel) oil are also high in saturated fat, as is cocoa butter. You'll find tropical oils in many snacks and in nondairy foods, such as coffee creamers and whipped toppings.

Another type of saturated fat, called *trans fats*, is produced when hydrogen is added to liquid oils to solidify them. Food manufacturers use trans fats because they extend shelf life. You can't see them, because they're hidden in many processed foods and in just about every food that contains shortening. Research shows that trans fats can raise LDL cholesterol, lower HDL ("good") cholesterol, and raise the risk of clots, which can block arteries and cause strokes.

This information is especially relevant when it comes to packaged gluten-free foods. To avoid trans fats, check any gluten-free product's ingredients list for the words *hydrogenated* or *partially hydrogenated*. If you see either of them, put the product back on the shelf and walk on by!

THE GOOD (UNSATURATED) FATS

In general, unsaturated fat—mostly in oils from plants—is liquid at room temperature and thickens when refrigerated. There are three basic types of unsaturated fats: monounsaturated fats (MUFAs), polyunsaturated fats, and omega-3 fatty acids.

MUFAs are found in olives, nuts, and seeds, as well as their oils. Studies show that a MUFA-rich diet improves blood cholesterol levels, which reduces heart disease risk and may benefit insulin levels and blood sugar control. Research also suggests that a MUFA-rich diet can ease chronic inflammation, boost brain function, and reduce cancer risk (learn more about these benefits on page 10). Most important of all, it helps the body metabolize a dangerous type of abdominal fat that we'll discuss in more detail on the next page. Due to this property, MUFAs are the cornerstone of the Flat Belly Diet, and we'll spend a good portion of this chapter showing you which foods offer the best sources of this precious healthy fat. That said, there are still two more types of beneficial fats that you should aim to eat more of.

Polyunsaturated fats are mainly in vegetable oils such as safflower, sunflower, sesame, soybean, and corn oils. Omega-3s are an exceptionally healthy type of polyunsaturated fat found mostly in fat-rich seafood, such as salmon, albacore tuna, herring, and mackerel. These special fats appear to reduce the risk of coronary artery disease and may help lower blood pressure and protect against irregular heartbeats. If you'd rather get a root canal than eat the recommended two fish meals a week, then you can get your dose of omega-3 fatty acids from walnuts, flaxseeds, or flaxseed oil instead.

Now that you know the difference between good and bad dietary fats, let's turn our attention to another type of fat. This type isn't in your food; it's in *you*.

The Big Bad Belly

Yes, belly fat puts a damper on bathing suit season. But the truth is, unlike run-of-the-mill butt, hip, or batwing-under-the-arm fat, belly fat can be life threatening.

To understand why, you first have to know that we have two types of body fat. *Subcutaneous fat* is the fat you can see, the inch (or more) you can pinch. For the most part, it's everywhere—even the soles of your feet have it.

Visceral fat is packed deep in your torso, wrapping itself around your heart, liver, and other major organs. Even relatively thin people can have too much visceral fat. You just can't see it, which is why it is sometimes referred to as "hidden" belly fat. To help you figure out if you've got too much, the National Institutes of Health (NIH) recommends the following belly cutoff point: A waist measurement of above 35 inches for women and 40 inches for men is an unhealthy sign of excess visceral fat.

Whether hidden or right out front, belly fat doesn't just sit there. It's alive. Visceral fat functions like a separate organ, releasing stress hormones that can be harmful to your body. Visceral fat has been linked to high blood pressure, stroke, heart disease, and diabetes, among other adverse health conditions.

In fact, belly fat may have a greater impact on the cardiovascular health of older women than overall obesity, according to a study published in *Circulation: Journal of the American Heart Association*. Danish researchers found that women with excessive belly fat had a greater risk of atherosclerosis than those whose fat was stored mostly in their hips, thighs, and buttocks. And in research published in the medical journal *The Lancet*, doctors concluded that waist measurement is a more accurate forecaster of heart attacks than body mass index (BMI)!

Worse yet, researchers increasingly suspect that visceral fat is involved in inflammatory processes associated with many chronic diseases. For example, a study conducted at the Washington University School of Medicine found that fat cells in the abdomen secrete molecules that increase inflammation. And an animal study conducted by the University of Michigan Department of Internal Medicine directly linked visceral fat, inflammation, and atherosclerosis (which in humans sets the stage for most heart attacks and strokes).

But don't worry—there are some strong rays of hope in all this grim news. As you'll see below, there's compelling evidence that MUFAs not only reduce the accumulation of visceral fat, they actually target belly fat. The best news of all? They do so deliciously.

BMI: THE BASICS

Body mass index (BMI) is a measure of body fat based on height and weight. While BMI does not measure body fat directly, it's a simple and reliable way to assess whether the amount of body fat a person carries may lead to health problems.

A BMI of 18.5 to 24.9 is considered healthy for both women and men. According to the National Heart, Lung, and Blood Institute, a BMI of 25.0 to 29.9 indicates a person is overweight, and 30 or more indicates obesity. (A BMI below 18.5 is considered underweight.)

Knowing your BMI can help you determine if you are at a healthy weight. To calculate your BMI, multiply your weight in pounds by 703. Divide that number by your height in inches. Then divide that number by your height in inches again.

Is your BMI higher than is healthy? Don't let it throw you. Now that you're on the path to better health and a slimmer figure, use that number as your motivation to get fit.

THE TOP 5 REASONS FOR A BIG BELLY

Why do some people (maybe you?) store more fat deep in their bellies, while others carry it on their hips and thighs? Extra calories and a sofa-spud lifestyle aren't the only reasons. These five factors play key roles:

1. **Your genetic makeup.** Your genes are from 30 to 60 percent responsible for where your body stores fat. (But lifestyle plays a big role in how much you store there.)
2. **Your age.** While most of us gain fat all over as we age, the accumulation of visceral fat seems to pick up with the years. In one Canadian study of 174 women, those approaching their 50th birthdays had twice as much visceral fat as those in their twenties, even though the older women weighed only 12 to 15 pounds more. Similar results have been found in men.
3. **Your gender.** In general, humans store 10 to 15 percent of their total body fat as visceral fat. But men store twice as much of their fat deep in their bellies as premenopausal women do.
4. **Menopause.** Thanks to changing hormones, a woman's body burns 30 percent less fat and stores more deep belly fat after menopause. One Syracuse University study of 54 postmenopausal women found that 20 to 30 percent of their total body fat was visceral fat.

5. **Food choices.** Diets high in saturated fats, found in fatty meats and full-fat dairy products, have been linked with higher levels of visceral fat. Brazilian researchers have found that trans fats—fats found in fast foods and many packaged foods—seem to concentrate in visceral fat. In contrast, MUFA-rich diets (like Flat Belly Diet Gluten-Free) discourage the formation of this deep belly fat.

"Medicine" from the Mediterranean

Roughly a half century ago, researcher Ancel Keys and his colleagues were studying the epidemic levels of heart disease in the United States. At the time of Keys's research, Greece, and especially the island of Crete, had the highest life expectancy in the world. It also had the lowest rate of coronary heart disease—80 to 90 percent lower than the United States at that time—even though its citizens consumed an unusually high amount of fat, mainly from olive oil.

Their long-term studies found that people live longer, healthier lives and weigh less when their diets include substantial amounts of fruits, veggies, and legumes; nuts, olives, and olive oil (MUFAs!); and whole grains, lots of fish, and very little red meat. That's the basic dietary pattern for the famous and rigorously studied Mediterranean Diet, considered by many nutrition experts to be one of the healthiest—and zestiest—in the world.

Keys's research put olive oil on the map, nutritionally speaking. It was the original MUFA rock star. Hundreds of studies have found that olive oil lowers levels of LDL cholesterol and triglycerides, lowers blood pressure, and raises HDL cholesterol. But MUFAs are found in many other foods, including almonds, guacamole, and dark chocolate—the same kinds of foods you may have banned in the past while trying to lose weight.

Meanwhile, evidence of MUFAs' unique heart-healthy powers continues to pile up:

○ A Pennsylvania State University study found that a MUFA-rich diet lowered LDL cholesterol by an average of 14 percent in 4 weeks, with no reduction of HDL cholesterol.

○ Canadian scientists found that a diet substituting MUFAs for some carbohydrates (but not reducing overall calorie intake) improved blood triglyceride levels and other markers for cardiovascular disease.

○ Researchers at Johns Hopkins University observed that diets low in saturated fat and rich in MUFAs lowered blood pressure and improved blood fat levels.

With its dazzling and delicious array of fruits and vegetables, nuts and seeds, and oils, Flat Belly Diet Gluten-Free is modeled on the Mediterranean Diet. While there are regional variations on this ultrahealthy way of eating (many countries border the Mediterranean Sea), all traditional Mediterranean diets include more plant foods and less animal protein. What the Mediterranean Diet is not low in: total fat. But most of the fat is in the form of heart-protective, belly-flattening MUFAs.

Because the Mediterranean way of eating is healthy, satisfying, and mouthwateringly delicious, many weight loss plans have gone Mediterranean. Flat Belly Diet Gluten-Free departs from the traditional Mediterranean Diet in two ways.

1. It "prescribes" a specific amount of MUFAs (including, but not limited to, olive oil) at each meal. That's because an ever-expanding body of research continues to find that MUFAs benefit both health and weight.
2. It removes whole grains that contain gluten. However, you can still eat gluten-free grains and grain products. You'll learn more about those in Chapter 2.

Get Ready for the Belly Revolution!

A healthier heart, a reduced risk of chronic diseases, protection against breast cancer . . . you can reap all these benefits, just from eating tasty foods that are naturally high in MUFAs. Add one more benefit to the list: A growing body of research singles out MUFAs as being particularly effective at fighting excess fat. This isn't just good news for the bikini in the back of your dresser drawer. Obesity is the common risk factor among many of the health conditions discussed thus far, including heart disease and diabetes.

The idea that eating fat may help you lose fat isn't entirely new. In the mid-1990s, while many of us were munching our fat-free cookies, Pennsylvania State University researchers assigned 53 overweight women and men to either a low-fat diet packed with carbs or a higher-fat diet with plenty of MUFAs. Compared to the carb eaters, the MUFA group saw a 20 percent greater reduction in visceral fat!

A few years later, researchers at Harvard-affiliated Brigham and Women's Hospital randomly assigned 101 overweight men and women to either a low-fat or Mediterranean-style diet. After 18 months, the low-fat group averaged a 6-pound weight gain, while the Mediterranean group lost an average of 9 pounds.

But the study that caught our eye here at *Prevention* was a small 2007 study published in the journal *Diabetes Care*, which dropped this bombshell: While

(continued on page 12)

EVEN MORE MUFA POWER

When it comes to MUFAs' health benefits, heart protection is just the beginning. A steady stream of research studies link MUFAs to reduced rates of other serious diseases, including:

Type 2 Diabetes

Being overweight and carrying belly fat are big risk factors. Research points to MUFAs in particular as potential superheroes for controlling blood sugar, reducing insulin resistance, and fighting visceral fat, the dangerous kind found deep in the abdomen that's strongly associated with prediabetes and diabetes.

A MUFA-rich diet benefited people with type 2 diabetes, according to a report published in the *American Journal of Clinical Nutrition*, by significantly improving their blood glucose profiles while reducing LDL cholesterol and triglycerides and significantly raising HDL cholesterol. In another study, Indiana University researchers found that treating obese people with type 2 diabetes with a MUFA-enriched weight-reducing diet resulted not only in weight loss, but also reductions in total cholesterol and triglyceride levels. These improvements remained even for those who eventually regained the weight.

Metabolic Syndrome

Affecting an estimated 50 million Americans, metabolic syndrome is characterized by a group of risk factors including abdominal obesity (a.k.a. belly fat); high blood pressure; blood-fat disorders such as high LDL, high triglycerides, and low HDL; insulin resistance; and glucose intolerance. Not surprisingly, metabolic syndrome increases risks of coronary heart disease, stroke, and type 2 diabetes.

MUFAs can help protect against metabolic syndrome, a review published in the *Journal of Clinical Nutrition* found. The review summarized findings that a MUFA-rich diet improves insulin sensitivity and blood lipid levels. And a study at Columbia University College of Physicians and Scientists concluded that treating people with metabolic syndrome by replacing saturated fat with MUFAs significantly reduced the risk of coronary heart disease. In fact, it worked better than replacing saturated fat with carbohydrates.

Chronic Inflammation

The body's natural defensive response to injury and illness, inflammation is a complex biological process that can run amok. If it becomes chronic, it can lead to atherosclerosis, rheumatoid arthritis, and asthma, among other diseases.

MUFAs work synergistically with other nutrients, such as antioxidants, to produce anti-inflammatory substances that can help reduce the severity of inflammatory symptoms in diseases like rheumatoid arthritis and asthma. Another study conducted in Italy linked Mediterranean diets featuring MUFA-rich foods with significantly lower concentrations of inflammatory markers in the blood.

Breast Cancer

In a study conducted in the Canary Islands, women with the most MUFAs in their diets had 48 percent less chance of breast cancer than those whose consumption was lowest. Another study, published in the *Annals of Oncology*, found that oleic acid, a type of MUFA abundant in olive oil, avocados, and nuts, enhanced the ability of cancer-fighting drugs to stop the growth of aggressive, treatment-resistant cancer cells.

In a Swedish study examining data on more than 61,000 mostly postmenopausal women, results were truly dramatic. Researchers found an inverse association between MUFAs and cancer risk—with 45 percent reduction in the risk of developing breast cancer for each 10-gram increment of MUFAs consumed daily.

Brain Function

Italian studies have found that a high intake of MUFAs as part of a Mediterranean diet offers great protection against age-related cognitive decline. And an American study published in the *Annals of Neurology* concluded that the more faithfully participants from the Washington Heights-Inwood Columbia Aging Project followed a MUFA-rich Mediterranean diet, the lower their incidence of Alzheimer's disease. Subjects who stuck closest to the diet had 40 percent less chance of developing Alzheimer's than those who adhered to it the least.

diets rich in carbs or saturated fats lead to fat deposits around the middle, a high-MUFA diet with the same number of calories actually prevents the accumulation of visceral belly fat!

That's right—MUFAs seem to actually discourage the storage of new belly fat. In another groundbreaking 2007 study, researchers in Spain tracked 59 people who followed either a high-carbohydrate eating plan or one that was high in saturated or monounsaturated fats. After 4 weeks, none of the participants lost or gained weight. But amazingly, their body fat actually redistributed itself. The MUFA group's belly fat shrank, while the carb group lost fat in their lower bodies, but gained fat in their bellies.

Researchers are still working to identify the exact metabolic process behind the MUFA weight loss. But looking at the results, it's as if eating a MUFA-rich diet gives your body a new set of instructions: Lose belly fat!

Now that you're clued in to the science behind Flat Belly Diet Gluten-Free, let's start talking about what to eat!

"DO I HAVE TO WORK OUT?"

Nope. That's what makes Flat Belly Diet Gluten-Free unique: To reap the benefits, you don't even have to break a sweat.

Don't get us wrong. We're all for regular exercise. It's an integral part of a healthy lifestyle and will make it easier for you to keep those lost pounds from coming back. But if you're not ready to start exercising regularly, we understand. You've got enough on your plate with the food part of the plan. (You really do. Have you checked out the pictures of the food yet?) There's plenty of time to reevaluate the decision to exercise 32 days from now, when you've dropped weight and gained energy. What's important is that you're taking steps to reduce your belly fat today.

If you do exercise, you'll almost certainly see results faster, as well as gain secondary benefits like improved cardiovascular health and strong, more toned muscles. But whether you work out or not, you can still expect to shrink your belly—and lose both subcutaneous and visceral fat—by simply following the eating plan alone. We predict that you'll be ready to lace up your walking shoes 32 days from now!

The MUFA Rock Stars

Now for the moment you've been waiting for: the five core foods of the Flat Belly Diet Gluten-Free. There are five categories of MUFAs: oils, olives, nuts and seeds, avocados, and (yum!) dark chocolate. In Chapter 3, we'll give you dozens of practical tips on how to buy, store, and use them to maximize their taste and health benefits. For now, here's a snapshot of each.

OILS: LIQUID MUFA GOLD

As we mentioned, olive oil is the original MUFA superstar. The ancient Greek poet Homer described it as liquid gold.

Extra-virgin olive oil is loaded with polyphenols—phytochemicals shown in studies to be potent antioxidants. In a 2010 study of 20 people with metabolic syndrome, Spanish researchers found that the oil's phenol compounds may "switch off" genes that promote heart-threatening inflammation.

During the two-phase study, the volunteers followed the same low-fat, carbohydrate-rich diet. Only the breakfasts were different. The first breakfast contained high-phenol virgin olive oil. After a 6-week "washout" period, in which they were instructed to not take vitamins, soy supplements, or any drugs, they consumed the other breakfast, made with low-phenol olive oil.

After each breakfast phase, the researchers tracked the expression of more than 15,000 human genes in the volunteers' blood cells. Consuming the phenol-rich olive oil "switched off" 79 genes, many of which have been linked to obesity, high blood-fat levels, diabetes, and heart disease, the study found. Further, several of those turned-down genes are known to promote inflammation and so may "cool off" the inflammation that accompanies metabolic syndrome.

Beyond olive oil, there are other tasty MUFA-rich oils you'll want to try.

Flaxseed and walnut oils are both rich sources of alpha-linolenic acid, which converts to omega-3 fatty acids in the body. Studies have shown that omega-3 fatty acids can raise beneficial HDL cholesterol, lower harmful LDL cholesterol, prevent abnormal heart rhythms, lower your risk of heart disease, and inhibit the development of blood clots.

Walnut oil is also high in the phytochemical ellagic acid, a powerful antioxidant that counters the effects of cell-damaging free radicals, which contribute to cancer and other diseases.

Canola, sesame, sunflower, and safflower oils are rich in vitamin E. They're excellent for roasting and sautéing (canola oil), stir-frying (sesame oil), and dressing salads (safflower and sunflower oils).

OLIVES: TINY BUT TASTY

Whether you opt for black or green olives or tapenade—the tangy spread made from olives, olive oil, garlic, and herbs—these luscious, MUFA-rich fruits cause body-chemistry changes that usher dangerous visceral fat out.

MEN: GET READY FOR FLAT ABS!

Women may be Venusians while men come from Mars, and the way they gain weight is different, too. Women tend to put the weight on their hips, thighs, and butt, while men concentrate the flab in just one place—their belly!

Unfortunately, hitting the gym more often won't necessarily help men shed that dangerous, heart-threatening abdominal fat, put on by pounding drinks with the guys and midnight junk food binges. Neither will simply cutting calories. That spare tire isn't just unsightly—it can increase a man's risk of heart disease, stroke, type 2 diabetes, sleep apnea, and even certain cancers.

What will help: loading up on gut-slimming, stomach-satisfying MUFAs. And with the help of non-gluten-containing grains and gluten-free foods, you won't miss the wheat, only the weight. What you will gain is renewed energy and the opportunity to see your abs again. (We don't force you to exercise, but if you're hitting the gym anyway, eating the flat-belly, gluten-free way will help you get fit faster.)

Welcome to a gluten-free weight loss plan that actually features food you want to eat, and plenty of it. Whether you're a guy with celiac disease or gluten sensitivity, Flat Belly Diet Gluten-Free can work wonders. The best part: Because men are typically heavier and more muscular than women, they get to eat more—a 1,600-calorie Jumpstart and 2,000 calories during the diet phase of the plan.

Yes, you must drink the Sassy Water during the Jumpstart phase. Or, for a spicy metabolism-boosting alternative, try our Fire Water recipe. Both are listed on page 19.

Olives contain antioxidants called polyphenols, which research suggests help to reduce inflammation in the blood vessels, improving cholesterol and triglyceride levels. They're also a good source of iron, vitamin E, copper (a mineral that protects your nerves, thyroid, and connective tissue), and fiber (to regulate your digestive system, help control blood sugar levels, and manage blood cholesterol).

NUTS AND SEEDS: FLAVORFUL AND FIBER-FULL

Nuts and seeds (walnuts, pistachios, sunflower seeds, and more) are packed with MUFAs and key nutrients—and while they help flatten your belly, they protect your health.

- **Walnuts.** They have the highest content of omega-3s of any nut and may help clear plaque from your arteries. Researchers in Spain gave two groups of people a heart-healthy diet that differed in just one respect: One diet included 8 to 13 walnuts a day. After 4 weeks, the walnut eaters had 64 percent stronger artery-pumping action and 20 percent less gunky molecules that initiate atherosclerotic plaque.

- **Pistachios.** Pennsylvania State University researchers found that adults who got 20 percent of their calories from pistachios (that's about ½ cup for an 1,800-calorie diet) reduced LDL cholesterol by 12 percent.

- **Sunflower seeds.** These seeds happen to be rich in linoleic acid. Women who had the highest intakes of this substance had a 23 percent lower risk of heart disease, compared with those with the lowest intakes. For a full list of MUFA-licious nuts and seeds, turn to Appendix B, Your MUFA Serving Chart, on page 294.

All this, and these fat-packed treats may help you manage your weight, too. Several studies have associated two or more servings of nuts a week with lower weight and avoidance of weight gain. For example, in a 2010 study, researchers at Beth Israel Deaconess Medical Center reported that people who ate walnuts at breakfast felt fuller, which made it easier for them to eat less at lunch.

Researchers think that the fiber and protein in nuts help make you feel full longer, so you're less hungry and eat less at your next meal. And there's some evidence that nuts may affect metabolism in a way that compensates for the high calories they contain.

AVOCADOS: BUTTERY GOODNESS

If you haven't enjoyed a salad studded with chunks of this pale green fruit or savored the thick, creamy guacamole dip made from it, you're in for a treat! The avocado's soft texture and mild, delicate, nutlike flavor make it a tasty and versatile addition to just about any dish. Slice it onto a sandwich. Enjoy it "naked," dressed with olive oil and balsamic vinegar. And go ahead—blend some into your favorite smoothie! No matter how you slice it, smooth, creamy avocados are packed with fat-fighting MUFAs and some pretty tasty health benefits.

Avocados are loaded with a natural, plant-based fat called beta-sitosterol, which has been found to reduce the amount of cholesterol absorbed from food. And in an Ohio State University study, adding 3 tablespoons of avocado to salsas and salads was shown to more than double the volunteers' absorption of carotenoids—antioxidants linked to lower risk of heart disease and macular degeneration, a leading cause of blindness.

Avocados are also high in fiber, a good source of the antioxidant vitamin E, the heart-protective B vitamin folate, and the mineral potassium, which is critical for nerve impulse transmission, muscle contraction, and heart function. Avocados also provide a fair amount of magnesium, which helps the body metabolize carbohydrates and fats.

DARK CHOCOLATE: MUFA-LICIOUS!

This is definitely the most decadent, delicious way to indulge your tastebuds while flattening your belly and lowering your blood pressure. Dark chocolate is packed with heart-healthy *flavonoids*—natural compounds that relax blood vessels, thereby lowering blood pressure, according to recent studies. In 2011, Harvard researchers found that eating a small square of dark chocolate each day can help lower blood pressure for people with hypertension.

The study analyzed 24 chocolate studies involving 1,106 people. It found that dark chocolate, the kind that contains at least 50 to 70 percent cocoa (or cacao, as it's sometimes referred to on packaging), lowered blood pressure in everyone, but most notably in those with high blood pressure. Researchers also found that chocolate increased insulin sensitivity, which can help lower diabetes risk, and found some evidence for a significant increase in good HDL cholesterol and a small reduction in bad LDL cholesterol.

But why the dark stuff over white or milk chocolate? Because chocolate with a higher proportion of cocoa solids, like unsweetened or dark chocolate, contains more flavonoids, the Harvard study said. For example, an ounce of dark chocolate contains 46 to 61 milligrams of the flavonoid catechin. The same amount of milk chocolate contains 15 to 16 milligrams. Dark chocolate also contains important minerals including copper, magnesium, potassium, calcium, and iron.

The Flat Belly Gluten-Free Food Plan

Now that you know what you'll eat, it's time to learn how to work the plan. The Flat Belly Diet Gluten-Free food plan consists of two phases: the Jumpstart and the plan itself. Each phase has been modified from the original to be gluten free, and you'll enjoy satisfying amounts of gluten-free grains and products on both. You'll learn the ins and outs of avoiding gluten, both at home and while dining out, in Chapter 2. For now, let's go over the nuts and bolts of the basic plan.

The Jumpstart will help you shed bloat, tame gas, and get your motivation and weight loss rolling. Post-Jumpstart, you'll continue to shed belly and body fat—and eat more calories, too. Here's a cheat sheet to make each phase crystal clear.

PHASE 1: THE 4-DAY ANTI-BLOAT JUMPSTART

4 days, four meals, 1,200 calories/day for women or 1,600 calories/day for men

- Follow the plan exactly.
- Avoid the bad guys of bloat.
- After each meal, take a 5-minute walk.
- Drink a 2-liter pitcher of Sassy Water or Fire Water every day.

Here's a happy thought: You're 4 days away from a flatter belly! The Jumpstart sparks your motivation and makes you feel sleeker and slimmer from the get-go. As you set aside food and beverages that can cause bloat, water retention, and GI irritation (namely, salty and fried foods, and carbonated and caffeinated beverages), your belly will flatten dramatically as your system releases extra fluid and trapped air. You'll also prime your body to shed belly fat. Here's what you'll do for the next 4 days.

Follow the plan exactly. You'll eat four times a day on the Jumpstart plan—three meals plus a fruity, satisfying smoothie for women, or four 400-calorie meals for men. Eat all four meals, even if you're not used to eating breakfast. You'll soon get into the rhythm of eating four times a day, or roughly every 3 to 4 hours.

Avoid the bad guys of bloat. There are a number of foods you probably eat every day that actually encourage that bloated, uncomfortable feeling wedging itself between you and your favorite pair of jeans. Here's the list of foods you need to say farewell to for the next 4 days:

- **Bulky raw veggies.** Carrots, beets, and other bulky veggies are good for you, and yes, you *can* eat them—just cook them rather than consuming them raw. Veggies with a lot of volume can expand your GI tract—exactly what you want to avoid. On the Jumpstart plan, make the steamer your friend.

- **Foods that produce gas.** The goal is to de-bloat your belly, so it only makes sense to steer clear of foods that can puff up your GI tract with gas. These include broccoli, cauliflower, Brussels sprouts, legumes, citrus fruits, onions, and peppers.

- **Fried foods.** Your GI tract digests fat-laden foods more slowly, which can lead to bloat. Pass them up and you'll feel slimmer and sleeker. Especially avoid foods that are both fatty and deep-fried.

- **Spicy foods.** Avoiding them will help prevent the release of stomach acid, which can cause bloating and irritation. So limit your use of black pepper, chili powder, hot sauces, and vinegar. Ditto for sweet spices such as cloves and nutmeg, and condiments such as ketchup, horseradish, and barbeque sauce.

- **Certain sugar substitutes.** Think you can sneak in a few low-calorie or low-carb gluten-free cookies? Don't chance it. Some of these diet products (including candies, sugar-free mints, and energy bars) contain the sugar alcohols xylitol and manitol, which can cause bloating and painful gas if you eat too much of them. Check a food's ingredient label to find them.

- **Chewing gum.** If you're chomping to quell a craving, give it up for these few days. Along with the flavor, you're swallowing air—lots of it. That air can get trapped in your GI tract, and your belly will show it. Plus, sugar-free gum may also contain those gas-producing sugar alcohols mentioned above.

○ **Gas-producing beverages.** Fizzy drinks like soda will bloat your belly (where else are those bubbles to go?). And coffee, tea, hot cocoa, acidic fruit juices, and alcohol can irritate your GI tract, leading to abdominal bloating. You may be wondering what's left to drink, but don't worry, we'll get to that soon!

After each meal, take a 5-minute walk. We're talking a stroll around the block or even inside your office building. When you move, you help your body release air trapped in your GI tract, relieving pressure and bloating. And yes, you can walk more if you want to!

Drink a 2-liter pitcher of Sassy Water or Fire Water every day. Diet or no, your body needs to stay hydrated, and water is better than coffee (loaded with caffeine), diet soda (packed with bubbles), or juice (packed with calories). Our drinks, though, are quite a treat—a flavorful blend of citrus, cucumber, mint, and spices stirred up into 2 liters of refreshing, revitalizing water.

SASSIFY YOURSELF

Sassy Water—a blend of water, herbs, and cool, refreshing cucumber—is a tasty, healthy substitute for belly-bloating carbonated diet beverages. You don't have to drink it after the Jumpstart phase of the diet, but you can if you want—many Flat Belly dieters love it! Make a fresh batch each day and feel free to omit any ingredients you don't like. Or, try our spicier take on this refreshing, hydrating, metabolism-boosting beverage.

Sassy Water

2 liters water (about 8½ cups)
1 teaspoon grated fresh ginger
1 medium cucumber, peeled and thinly sliced

1 medium lemon, thinly sliced
12 fresh mint leaves

Fire Water

2 liters water
½ teaspoon grated fresh ginger
1 small cucumber, peeled and thinly sliced
1 lime, quartered, seeds removed

6 mint leaves
3 or 4 dashes gluten-free hot sauce (such as Frank's RedHot or Tabasco)

For both recipes, combine all of the ingredients in a large pitcher and chill in the refrigerator overnight, to let the flavors blend. A few tips:

○ Use any type of fresh mint, but don't substitute dried mint or mint extract—it will taste yucky in water. Ditto for the ginger—it must be fresh, not dry or ground.

JUMP TO IT! YOUR 4-DAY SHOPPING LIST

This will be a quick shopping trip—you'll be eating a limited number of foods during the 4-Day Anti-Bloat Jumpstart. These foods were specifically chosen to reduce bloating and flatulence, giving you immediate waist-slimming results while also kickstarting your weight loss. If the menu looks restrictive, don't worry: You'll be able to reintroduce your favorite foods after just 4 days.

Remember: Check labels before you buy. All grains, such as quinoa and brown rice, must be labeled "gluten free," as must all deli meats, herbs, and seasonings. These items may be produced in a facility that also makes gluten-containing products. To avoid cross-contamination, be sure to read all labels to ensure each product is gluten free (for more information about cross-contamination, see page 56).

PRODUCE

○ 1 pint blueberries

○ 2 pints grape tomatoes

○ 2 cups fresh or frozen green beans

○ 2 large red potatoes

○ 10-ounce bag baby carrots

○ 4 celery stalks

○ ½ pint cremini mushrooms

○ 1 large zucchini

○ 4 medium cucumbers

○ 4 medium lemons

DAIRY

○ ½ gallon lactose-free, fat-free milk

○ 1 package low-fat string cheese

○ 6-ounce fat-free strawberry yogurt

FROZEN FOODS

○ 10-ounce bag unsweetened strawberries

○ 10-ounce bag unsweetened peaches

- Strain the ingredients or just pour them into the glass. Feel free to snack on the cucumber—it'll cost you less than 25 calories.

- If you find the taste of Sassy Water or Fire Water too strong, prepare your pitcher in the morning instead of the night before, so the flavors won't be as intense. Or use smaller amounts of ginger, lemon, mint, or hot sauce.

DRY GOODS

- ☐ 12-ounce box whole grain gluten-free cereal
- ☐ 12-ounce box quinoa
- ☐ 14-ounce box instant brown rice
- ☐ 8-ounce can unsweetened pineapple chunks in pineapple juice
- ☐ 1 cup roasted or raw unsalted sunflower seeds, without shells
- ☐ 1 cup roasted or raw unsalted almonds
- ☐ 8-ounce bottle cold-pressed organic flaxseed oil
- ☐ 8-ounce bottle olive oil
- ☐ 15-ounce package raisins

SPICES

- ☐ 2-ounce bottle ground cinnamon
- ☐ 1 to 2 knuckles fresh ginger
- ☐ 2 bunches fresh mint

MEAT/SEAFOOD

- ☐ ½ pound organic low-sodium deli turkey breast
- ☐ ¼ pound tilapia
- ☐ 6 ounces organic boneless skinless chicken breast
- ☐ ¼ pound organic turkey breast cutlet
- ☐ 2 cans (3 ounces each) chunk light tuna in water

SALT-FREE SEASONINGS

- ☐ Original and Italian medley Mrs. Dash gluten-free, salt-free seasoning blends
- ☐ Fresh or dried: basil, bay leaf, cinnamon, curry powder, dill, ginger, lemon or lime juice, marjoram, mint, oregano, paprika, pepper, rosemary, sage, tarragon, or thyme

Note: Never purchase grains, seeds, or other foods from bulk bins as cross-contamination may occur.

Day 1

BREAKFAST

1 cup gluten-free cereal

1 cup fat-free milk

¼ cup roasted or raw unsalted sunflower seeds

2 tablespoons raisins

Glass of Sassy Water or Fire Water

LUNCH

3 ounces chunk light tuna in water

1 cup steamed baby carrots

1 reduced-fat string cheese

Glass of Sassy Water or Fire Water

SNACK

STRAWBERRY SMOOTHIE: In a blender, combine 1 cup fat-free milk and 1 cup frozen unsweetened strawberries. Blend for 1 minute, or until smooth. Transfer to a tall glass and stir in 1 tablespoon cold-pressed organic flaxseed oil or serve with 1 tablespoon sunflower or pumpkin seeds.

DINNER

4 ounces grilled cod

1 cup cremini mushrooms sautéed with 1 teaspoon olive oil

½ cup cooked brown rice

Glass of Sassy Water or Fire Water

DAILY NUTRITION TOTAL: 1,363 calories, 93 g protein, 153 g carbohydrates, 47 g total fat, 7.5 g saturated fat, 16 g fiber, 896 mg sodium

Day 2

BREAKFAST

QUINOA BREAKFAST SUNDAE: Mix ½ cup cooked quinoa with ½ cup fat-free strawberry yogurt. Sprinkle with cinnamon. In a parfait glass, layer quinoa-yogurt mixture with 1 cup blueberries. Top with 2 tablespoons chopped almonds.

Glass of Sassy Water or Fire Water

LUNCH

4 ounces low-sodium gluten-free deli turkey, rolled up

1 cup grape tomatoes

1 cup celery sticks

1 reduced-fat string cheese

Glass of Sassy Water or Fire Water

SNACK

PEACH SMOOTHIE: In a blender, combine 1 cup fat-free milk and 1 cup frozen unsweetened peaches. Blend for 1 minute, or until smooth. Transfer to a tall glass and stir in 1 tablespoon cold-pressed organic flaxseed oil, or serve with 1 tablespoon sunflower or pumpkin seeds.

DINNER

3 ounces grilled chicken breast

1 cup zucchini sautéed with 1 teaspoon olive oil

½ cup roasted red potatoes drizzled with 1 teaspoon olive oil

Glass of Sassy Water or Fire Water

DAILY NUTRITION TOTAL: 1,165 calories, 87 g protein, 121 g carbohydrates, 44 g total fat, 6.5 g saturated fat, 19 g fiber, 1,334 mg sodium

Day 3

BREAKFAST

1 cup gluten-free cereal

1 cup fat-free milk

4 ounces unsweetened pineapple chunks canned in juice, drained

1/4 cup roasted or raw unsalted sunflower seeds

Glass of Sassy Water or Fire Water

LUNCH

3 ounces chunk light tuna in water

1 cup grape tomatoes

1 cup celery sticks

1 reduced-fat string cheese

Glass of Sassy Water or Fire Water

SNACK

BLUEBERRY SMOOTHIE: In a blender, combine 1 cup fat-free milk and 1 cup blueberries. Blend for 1 minute, or until smooth. Transfer to a tall glass and stir in 1 tablespoon cold-pressed organic flaxseed oil, or serve with 1 tablespoon sunflower or pumpkin seeds.

DINNER

3 ounces grilled or baked turkey breast cutlet

1 cup steamed green beans

1/2 cup cooked brown rice

Glass of Sassy Water or Fire Water

DAILY NUTRITION TOTAL: 1,222 calories, 88 g protein, 135 g carbohydrates, 41 g total fat, 6 g saturated fat, 20 g fiber, 763 mg sodium

Day 4

BREAKFAST

1 cup gluten-free cereal

1 cup fat-free milk

1/4 cup almonds

2 tablespoons raisins

Glass of Sassy Water or Fire Water

LUNCH

4 ounces low-sodium gluten-free deli turkey, rolled up

1 cup steamed baby carrots

1 reduced-fat string cheese

Glass of Sassy Water or Fire Water

SNACK

PINEAPPLE SMOOTHIE: In a blender, combine 1 cup fat-free milk and 4 ounces canned pineapple chunks, drained. Blend for 1 minute, or until smooth. Transfer to a tall glass and stir in 1 tablespoon cold-pressed organic flaxseed oil, or serve with 1 tablespoon sunflower or pumpkin seeds.

DINNER

3 ounces grilled chicken breast

1 cup steamed green beans

1/4 cup roasted potatoes drizzled with 1 teaspoon olive oil

Glass of Sassy Water or Fire Water

DAILY NUTRITION TOTAL: 1,251 calories, 93 g protein, 147 g carbohydrates, 39 g total fat, 6 g saturated fat, 17 g fiber, 1,478 mg sodium

PHASE 2: THE 28-DAY PLAN

4 meals, 1,600 calories/day for women
5 meals, 2,000 calories/day for men

- Rule #1: Stick to 400 calories per meal.
- Rule #2: Never go more than 4 hours without eating.
- Rule #3: Eat a MUFA at every meal.

In your never-ending bid to slim your belly, you've lived on cabbage soup, sipped only shakes, or otherwise severely limited calories and/or eliminated entire food groups. But along with the weight, you lost a few other things, too. Like muscle, bone density, and your will to live. (We've all been there.)

Flat Belly Diet Gluten-Free is different. No gnawing hunger or feelings of deprivation, plenty of delicious choices, and guidelines as simple as they come.

Stick to 400 calories per meal. All Flat Belly Diet Gluten-Free meals and snacks—each containing one yummy MUFA and zero gluten—total about 400 calories; you eat three meals and one snack daily. This means that each day, you're consuming about 1,600 calories. That's how much it takes for a woman of average height, frame size, and activity level to get to and stay at her ideal body weight. Experts say that 1,600 calories is enough to keep up your energy and support your immune system. Because men are typically larger and more muscular, they eat five meals a day, for a total of 2,000 calories.

Eat every 4 hours. Waiting too long to eat can cause you to become so hungry (and irritable) that it's hard to think through the healthiest meal choice, let alone prepare one. You'll probably want to tear into the first thing you see and then reach for seconds. That's why you must eat every 4 hours while following this plan. Flat Belly Diet Gluten-Free is comprised of three meals, plus a snack (a fourth meal) that you can eat in the morning, afternoon, or evening—whenever it's most convenient for you. But by mandating a meal (or snack) every 4 hours, you ensure your hunger never gets the best of you.

Add a MUFA to every meal. From almonds to peanut butter, olive oil to avocados, you've got lots of delicious choices. (No, we didn't forget the dark chocolate!) Feel free to substitute one MUFA for another as long as the calorie counts are nearly equivalent. For example, you can exchange almond butter (200 calories) for semisweet chocolate chips (207).

So let's take stock: You're eating 1,600 or 2,000 calories a day, you're eating every few hours, and you're eating yummy stuff like Almond Waffles with Tropical Fruit Salsa, Cider Pork Chops with Walnuts and Apples, and Dark Chocolate Fudge Pops. Outstanding!

Look Before You Cook

In general, using this book is pretty simple: Select a dish and get cooking! That said, the guidelines and tips below can help you enjoy this flavorful fare—and maximize your weight loss—in a safe and healthy manner.

- For recipes that fall under 400 calories, check the "Make It a Flat Belly Diet Meal" information at the bottom of the page for suggested accompaniments. Calorie values for those foods are noted in parentheses.

- If you don't care for those suggestions, opt for similar foods in the appropriate calorie range.

- Try to avoid having two MUFA servings in the same meal because that can make it tricky to stick to 400 calories per meal. To ensure the right balance of nutrition, flavor, and adherence to gluten-free guidelines, sometimes we do provide recipes that use two MUFAs, but we've done the legwork to ensure you're getting just the right amount of calories.

- If you're a vegetarian or simply prefer to eat less meat, you'll find plenty of meatless recipes to choose from. Also, feel free to use soy-based meat substitutes in recipes that include meat, poultry, or seafood—but always check labels to make sure those products are gluten free.

- If you have been diagnosed with celiac disease or non-celiac gluten sensitivity, share the program with your doctor or dietitian before starting, to make sure it's the right choice for you.

- If you are allergic to any of the key MUFA foods or have high blood pressure, type 2 diabetes, or some other chronic condition for which you are taking medication or following a special diet, get the green light from your doctor before you start the Flat Belly Diet Gluten-Free plan (or any food plan, for that matter).

If You're New to the Flat Belly Diet . . .

Welcome! As we mentioned, you'll get the particulars on making the Flat Belly Diet a gluten-free program in the next chapter. And we've made things easy for you by including Your 14-Day Meal Plan in Appendix A on page 286 so you can get the hang of the rules and rhythm of the diet. (You're also free to swap meals in and out, depending on your preferences, since they're all 400 calories each.)

Or, if you'd rather, build your own Flat Belly meals. Just pick your MUFA from Appendix B on page 294 and use the following simple formula:

If your MUFA is nuts, seeds, or oil, add:

- 3 ounces lean protein
- 2 cups raw or steamed veggies
- ½ cup cooked gluten-free grain, such as quinoa, buckwheat, or brown rice, *or* 1 slice gluten-free bread, 1 gluten-free tortilla, or half of a gluten-free pita *or* 1 cup fruit

    Example: 1 gluten-free pita filled with 3 ounces grilled chicken cubed and covered with 2 tablespoons tahini (sesame seed paste) and 2 cups mixed salad greens

If your MUFA is avocado or olives, pair it with:

- 3 ounces lean protein *or* 2 ounces lean protein plus 1 dairy (such as 1 slice cheese *or* ¼ cup shredded or crumbled cheese)
- 2 cups raw or steamed veggies
- 1 cup starchy veggies (beans, corn, peas, potatoes) *or* 1 cup cooked gluten-free grain (such as brown or wild rice) *or* 2 gluten-free bread servings (such as a gluten-free pita, wrap, or English muffin)

    Example: 3 ounces chunk light tuna in water arranged on 2 cups field greens topped with ½ cup garbanzo beans, ½ cup peas, and ¼ cup avocado

If your MUFA is dark chocolate, pair it with:

- 1 cup fruit plus 1 cup dairy such as fat-free milk, yogurt, ricotta, or cottage cheese *or* 1 serving grain such as gluten-free oatmeal or gluten-free waffle

    Example: ¼ cup dark chocolate chips mixed with 1 cup berries and 1 cup fat-free vanilla yogurt

With the nuts and bolts of Flat Belly Diet Gluten-Free firmly in mind, you're now ready to maximize your weight loss (and please your tastebuds) while eliminating gluten from your diet. No worries—it's simpler than you think!

How to Use This Cookbook

The *Flat Belly Diet! Gluten-Free Cookbook* gives you many different tools in your quest to lose belly fat safely and permanently. Now that you know how to follow the Flat Belly Diet plan, you may be wondering how all these pieces fit together.

MAKE IT A MEAL

This cookbook gives you over 150 recipes to choose from and enjoy on your weight loss journey. For any recipe that falls under 400 calories, you can look to our "Make It a Flat Belly Diet Meal" sections for suggestions on how to get enough calories into your meal. If you don't like our suggestions, you can always swap in your own favorites—but be careful to aim for the same calorie range as the accompaniments we have suggested.

MIX 'N' MATCH

The easiest part about following our 400-calorie rule is that you can use the recipes in this book to create a virtually endless combination of belly-flattening meals. We've provided Your 14-Day Meal Plan on page 286 to follow if you're just getting started with the Flat Belly lifestyle, but there's no need to stop there! Savor the Cinnamon-Raisin Breakfast Sandwich for lunch, if you prefer. Or cook up the Fiery Shrimp Tacos for a spicy breakfast. The power is in your hands and you'll get great results no matter how you mix and match your meals.

GO TOTALLY GLUTEN FREE

As you'll learn in Chapter 2, the recipes, ingredient lists, and other resources in this cookbook have been designed and written expressly for those who want to lose weight and need a gluten-free plan to get it done! For gluten-free newbies, we'll explain the very basics of gluten and how it can damage your health. For readers who know the drill, this means we'll periodically remind you to check labels, introduce you to new brands (check out our Resources section on page 299), and encourage you to eat fresh, wholesome food your body will love.

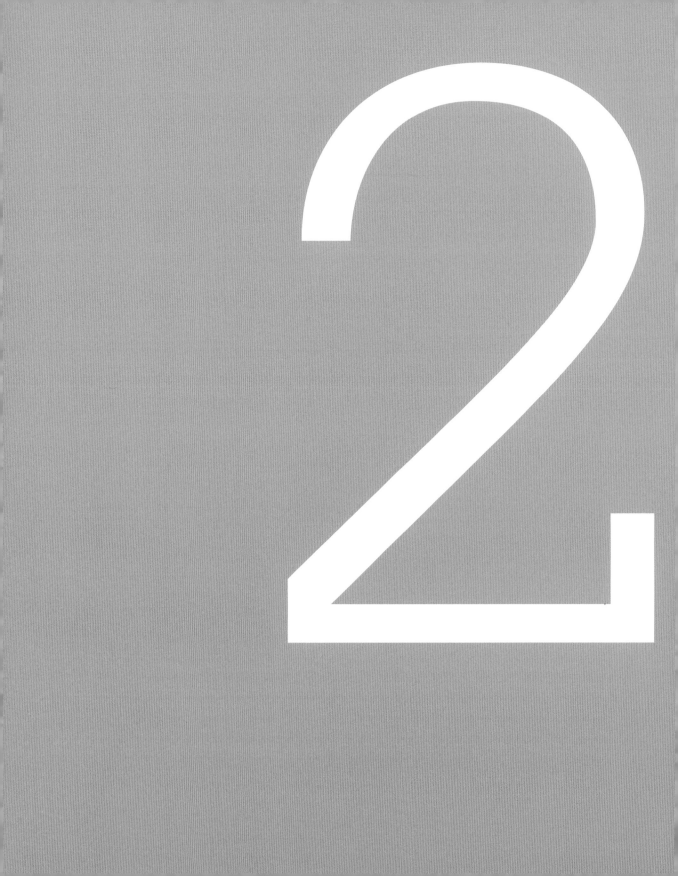

WHY EAT GLUTEN FREE?

If you've been diagnosed with celiac disease, you need to bid farewell to wheat, barley, rye, and triticale (a hybrid grain made from wheat and rye), because a gluten-free diet is the only treatment. But what if you *don't* have health issues that stem from ingesting gluten? Why would you voluntarily give up your English muffin or bagel at breakfast, your stromboli or slice of pizza at lunch, your plate of pasta at dinner?

Consider this: Many people have gluten sensitivities that go undiagnosed. Once you eliminate gluten, you may notice that many bothersome or uncomfortable symptoms you've simply learned to live with over time have lessened or virtually vanished.

It's difficult to dismiss the anecdotal evidence from those who never got a formal diagnosis of celiac disease, but—fed up with the cramps, bloating, moodiness, and mental fogginess—eliminated gluten from their diet in a bid to feel better. And many *do* feel better, physically and mentally. Many also report weight loss, along with more energy, brighter mood, and sharper mental focus. These individuals may in fact have non-celiac gluten sensitivity. If you suspect you have a gluten-related disorder, we strongly recommend you be tested by a doctor before starting a gluten-free diet to ensure you are taking every step to improve your overall health.

The gluten-free movement has exploded in recent years and the Flat Belly Diet Gluten-Free plan only increases its flavor, variety, and satisfaction. (All those yummy MUFAS!) This chapter explains how teaming the two eating styles can not only flatten your belly, but fight disease. But first, it's essential to understand the main reasons for following a gluten-free diet: celiac disease and non-celiac gluten sensitivity.

Celiac: A Gut-Wrenching Disease

Celiac disease affects just 1 percent of the population. But four times as many people have the condition today as compared to the 1950s, according to a 2012 study published in the *American Journal of Gastroenterology.* In another study published in 2010, researchers found that since the year 1974, the rate of celiac disease has doubled every 15 years. That research estimates that celiac disease may affect as many as 1 in every 133 Americans.

What gives? Why is this "rare" disease on the rise? One hypothesis among several: The grains we eat today are much richer in glutens than they were 70 or 80 years ago.

The bodies of people with celiac disease respond to gluten with a ferocious immune response that inflames the small intestine, damaging the millions of *villi* that carpet it. Normally, these slender, fingerlike projections that line the small intestine produce digestive enzymes and absorb nutrients. But if you looked at a piece of small intestine with celiac disease under a microscope, you would see flattened, stubby villi. This damage reduces their ability to make digestive enzymes and soak up nutrients.

People with celiac disease don't always know they have it because they may not feel sick. If they do feel sick (common symptoms include nausea, vomiting and diarrhea, abdominal pain and bloating, unintended weight loss, malnutrition, and anemia), they don't know celiac disease is the cause. Either way, their intestines are sustaining damage for as long as they continue to eat gluten-containing foods.

But that's not all. Undiagnosed celiac disease can lead to gastrointestinal cancers and some research has linked it to serious autoimmune disorders such as insulin-dependent (type 1) diabetes. In addition, the nutritional deficiencies that are a hallmark of the disease can precipitate a host of seemingly unrelated problems, including osteoporosis and, in pregnant women, fetal distress. (Low folic acid stores in moms can predispose unborn babies to serious neurological problems such as spina bifida.)

Celiac disease can be masked by—or mistaken for—other conditions, including allergies, colitis, irritable bowel syndrome, diabetes, thyroid disease, and garden-variety stress. Throw in a gluten-related food sensitivity such as lactose intolerance (due to those damaged villi), and doctors often throw up their hands. No wonder it takes an average of 11 years to be diagnosed!

The good news is that dietary changes can soothe your symptoms and reverse the damage that can lead to more serious illness.

If you suspect celiac disease (either because you're experiencing symptoms or you have a family history of the illness), schedule an appointment with a gastroenterologist pronto. These physicians, who specialize in problems of the stomach, intestines, gallbladder, and bile duct, typically have more experience with identifying and treating celiac and related diseases.

Once diagnosed, the only way to remain disease free is to swear off gluten. Because wheat is the primary source of gluten in the typical Western diet, any food made with wheat—from breakfast cereals to pizza, pasta, and bagels—must go. Fortunately, there are delicious swaps you can make for common gluten-containing ingredients, so you can still enjoy many of the foods you love. You will learn more about those in Chapter 3.

Most of the symptoms of celiac disease disappear within 6 months of totally eliminating gluten, although some people get relief within weeks. Even better news: Research suggests that in 5 years, the risk of intestinal cancers diminishes to match that of the general population.

TESTING FOR CELIAC DISEASE

Celiac disease is genetic—that is, your susceptibility is written in your chromosomes. But the disease isn't always inherited, and if it is, it can be triggered at any stage of life, from infancy to adulthood, by severe emotional stress, physical trauma, viral infection, pregnancy, or surgery.

The tests for genetic markers don't tell you if you have the disease; they're used to rule it out. For a positive diagnosis, the gold standard remains a small-bowel biopsy, in which doctors remove a tiny piece of your intestinal wall to analyze its texture and note any changes related to celiac disease.

Before you sign on for this outpatient procedure, however, you may want to ask your doctor about two relatively new blood tests: the antiendomysial antibody test and the tissue transglutaminase test. Both are designed to reveal the presence of antibodies related to celiac disease in your blood. To use one of the new diagnostic blood tests, you must be consuming gluten at the time of the test, or your results may not be accurate. If you test positive, your doctor will want to follow up with a small-bowel biopsy to make sure.

The "No-Man's-Land" of Gluten Sensitivity

Some people react to gluten in ways that experts don't yet fully understand. They show neither the autoimmune reactions that characterize celiac disease nor the allergic responses that typify wheat allergy. They're in the murky territory of non-celiac gluten sensitivity—one that's been called a no-man's-land of gluten-related problems.

Around 18 million Americans have gluten sensitivity, according to estimates from the University of Maryland's Center for Celiac Research. There's no official test for gluten sensitivity. Once your physician has determined that you do not have celiac disease or a wheat allergy, the next step is a gluten-elimination diet to see if symptoms resolve.

While some doctors have dismissed gluten sensitivity as an "all in your head" malady, there's compelling evidence that it's all too real. A recent University of Maryland study found that not only does gluten sensitivity exist, but it's also quite different from celiac disease—at least, in terms of how it works in your body.

In this study, a team led by Alessio Fasano, MD, looked for differences in immune reactions between people with celiac disease and people with gluten sensitivity. They conducted a series of lab tests and intestinal biopsies on 100 subjects in both groups, which revealed key physical differences: For one thing, people with gluten sensitivity generally don't have the damage to the small intestine that those with celiac disease have, nor do they have the specific markers in the blood used to diagnose celiac disease.

Researchers found that, compared to people with gluten sensitivity, those with celiac disease had a more severe immune response to gliadin, the toxic protein in gluten. This was indicated by higher levels of intestinal permeability, a condition in the GI tract that can lead to inflammation. In people with celiac disease, gliadin crosses the barrier between cells in the intestine, and the body attacks itself against what it sees as an invader: gluten.

While gluten sensitivity doesn't damage the intestine as celiac disease does, it can have a profoundly negative impact on physical, emotional, and mental well-being. Common symptoms include abdominal pain similar to irritable bowel syndrome, headaches, tingling, fatigue, muscle pain, skin rashes, and joint pain.

GETTING TO THE NITTY-GRITTY OF GLUTEN DISORDERS

Your belly is bloated, and you've got wicked stomach cramps. Or you're so fatigued, irritated, or mentally foggy you can't function. Your skin is breaking out, you're wheezing at work (but only at work), or you're unsteady on your feet.

Are you allergic to wheat? Do you have celiac disease or gluten sensitivity? Something rarer? More often than not, diagnosis and appropriate treatment can be a crapshoot. A recent proposal authored by heavyweights in the field of celiac disease aims to end that confusion. A group of 15 experts from seven countries is proposing a new classification system for the gluten-related disorders plaguing an increasing number of people worldwide, for reasons still unknown. The proposal (funded in part by a manufacturer of gluten-free products in Italy) defines a spectrum of illnesses based on the three kinds of immune defenses the human body mounts against gluten.

Allergic reactions. Symptoms occur minutes to hours after exposure to gluten, which could involve eating or breathing in wheat (the latter is known as baker's asthma). Allergic reactions can affect the skin, gastrointestinal tract, or respiratory tract, and symptoms can include hives, nasal and chest congestion, nausea, vomiting, and anaphylaxis.

Autoimmune reactions. Symptoms occur weeks to years after exposure to gluten. This category includes celiac disease; dermatitis herpetiformis; and gluten ataxia, which affects brain tissue, resulting in an unsteady gait and lack of motor control. Gluten may be the cause of ataxia in one-fifth of all those with the ailment, the report notes.

Immune-mediated reactions. Symptoms occur hours to days after gluten exposure. This category would include gluten sensitivity, in which people report the same symptoms as celiac disease, plus foggy thinking and mood swings, but test negative for telltale antibodies.

The proposal also spells out diagnostic criteria to help doctors determine which disorder their patients may have, if any, as well as specific treatments. Hopefully, gluten-related health problems will be caught more quickly, so the healing can begin.

GIVE GLUTEN-FREE "JUNK FOOD" A PASS

Eliminating wheat and gluten can result in a "snack gap"—suddenly, there are no cookies, pretzels, crackers, or snack bars. But, if you're eyeing stomach-friendly versions of these items in the gluten-free section of your supermarket, think twice before you buy. "Gluten free" doesn't always mean "healthy."

Gluten gives our favorite foods that special touch: It makes pizza dough stretchy, gives bread its spongy texture, and is used to thicken sauces and soups. Without it, food companies are forced to add extra fat and sugar to make up for the lack of texture and flavor. Previous studies that have analyzed the nutrient composition of packaged gluten-free products have found that these products tend to have high levels of fats (including unhealthy trans fats), sugars, and salt. What these packaged foods don't typically offer is fiber, which is essential to helping you maintain a healthy weight.

Other research has shown that people with celiac disease tend to compensate for the restrictions of a gluten-free diet by eating foods high in fat, sugar, and calories. Not surprisingly, they also consume excessive amounts of total and saturated fats overall. Not great for their health—or their waistlines, either.

Gluten-free foods tend to be pricier, too. (Six bucks for a box of cookies or crackers? Seriously?) Our suggestion: Enjoy gluten-free snacks as an occasional treat. But more often than not, opt for foods that are naturally gluten free, like those on the Flat Belly Diet Gluten-Free plan.

Mo' MUFA, No Gluten:
Two Great Plans in One

Gluten-free eating and the Mediterranean-inspired Flat Belly Diet are two great plans that taste great together. Both center on whole foods, deliver ample amounts of vital nutrients, and allow generous amounts of carbs from gluten-free grains, potatoes, and other natural foods. (And yes, you get dessert!) Combine the two eating styles, and you've got a plan that will peel off pounds—and belly fat—as it reduces your risk of diabetes, heart disease, and other maladies. If you have celiac disease or are sensitive to gluten, you'll likely find relief from your symptoms as you drop weight.

Although the core of the Flat Belly Diet Gluten-Free plan is those delicious, flavorful, and oh-so-satisfying MUFA foods, you'll be eating more (a lot more!). Here's a summary of the plan's building-block foods, which help you lose weight and protect your health.

HEARTY, GLUTEN-FREE GRAINS

Nutrition experts have long recommended that we swap refined carbs made with white flour for whole grains, and for good reasons. Whole grains are naturally low in fat, cholesterol free, and good sources of protein, fiber, minerals, vitamins, and other nutrients. And it has been well established by the scientific community that diets rich in whole grains are linked to a reduced risk of cardiovascular disease, diabetes, and some cancers.

Normally, when you think of whole grains, you think of wheat. But guess what? Gluten-free grains, also known as ancient or alternative grains, are also whole grains. (Technically, some are actually grasses, but you prepare and eat them like grains.) Historically, rice, corn, and potato were substitutes for grains that contain gluten. Today, other grains such as amaranth, buckwheat, flax, millet, teff, and quinoa offer more variety, nutrition, and flavor.

Ancient grains like amaranth, millet, and quinoa are often a richer source of nutrients than modern grains. For example, quinoa has been called a supergrain, because researchers have found that it can contain up to 50 percent more protein than common grains and higher levels of calcium, phosphorus, iron, and B vitamins. (See the "Nutrient Content of Common Gluten-Free Grains" chart on page 36.) Gluten-free whole grains are also good fiber sources.

That's excellent news, because research has found that gluten-free diets often run low in fiber.

You'll find alternative grains in the organic section of your supermarket or in natural foods stores. They're typically cooked and used like white rice and/or ground into flour. Their names may be unfamiliar to you, but humans around the world have been eating them for, well, forever. Amaranth and quinoa were the staple foods of the mighty Aztecs and Incas, respectively. Once the food of warriors, these grains now help us fight the diseases of modern civilization, obesity included. When you buy these grains at the store, you must ensure the packaging is labeled "gluten free" to avoid cross-contamination. For this reason, avoid buying from bulk bins.

Nutrient Content of Common Gluten-Free Grains
(per ½ cup serving, cooked)

GRAIN	FIBER, G	PROTEIN, G	IRON, MG	THIAMIN (VITAMIN B₁), MG	RIBOFLAVIN (VITAMIN B₂), MG	NIACIN (VITAMIN B₃), MG	FOLATE, MCG	ZINC, MG
Amaranth	2.5	4.5	2.6	~	~	0.3	27	1
Brown rice	1.8	2.5	0.4	0.095	0.025	1.5	3.9	0.61
Buckwheat groats	2.2	2.8	0.67	0.035	0.035	0.79	12	0.51
Millet	1.1	3	0.55	0.09	0.07	1.1	16.5	0.79
Oats	2.0	3	1	0.09	0.02	0.2	7	1.1
Quinoa	2.5	4	1.4	0.10	0.10	0.4	39	1.0
Teff		5		0.25	0.05	1.1	23	
Wild rice	1.5	3.5	0.50	0.05	0.05	1	21	1.1

Nutrient data for this listing was provided by USDA SR-21. Each "~" indicates a missing or incomplete value.

Wondering what they taste like and how to cook them? You'll find the answers in Chapter 3—check out our cheat sheet to help you get familiar with the many exotic (and delicious!) varieties, including preparation methods and serving suggestions.

EVEN MORE GOOD FATS

MUFA-rich foods such as walnuts, flaxseed, and olive and canola oils deliver a double dose of healthy fats: They're good sources of omega-3 and omega-6 fatty acids (fatty fish, too—see below). Among the benefits of these good fats:

They fight inflammation. Omega-3s cool chronic inflammation in the body, a major contributor to numerous chronic conditions, including insulin resistance and diabetes. Omega-6s suppress production of inflammation-related compounds, according to the American Heart Association. (The AHA recently recommended adding some omega-6s to our diets. While omega-6s have been demonized as a cause of inflammation, if you eat omega-3s and omega-6s in balance, both are beneficial.)

They reduce heart disease risk. A study at the Harvard School of Public Health found that women with diabetes who ate fish just once a week had a 40 percent lower risk of dying from heart disease than did women with diabetes who rarely ate fish.

You've no doubt heard about the heart-protecting powers of the omega-3 fats found in fatty, cold-water fish like salmon and mackerel (as well as in fish oil capsules). Worried about toxins in fish? It's true that fatty fish like salmon can accumulate chemical pollutants such as PCBs in their fat and skin, while leaner fish such as tuna can accumulate mercury in their flesh. But don't shy away from fin food—you need the good fats! To minimize your risk, eat two fish meals a week, eat a variety of fish, and favor types with lower levels of toxins, such as wild salmon (available in cans at the grocery store as well as in pricier fillets at the fish counter), mackerel, and herring.

Getting some of your omega-3s from walnuts, ground flaxseed, and flaxseed oil may help, too. These contain alpha-linoleic acid, which your body converts into the more potent omega-3 DHA, the type found in fish and fish oil capsules.

Dining Out, Flat Belly Style

If you enjoy dining out or are an on-the-run eater, Flat Belly Diet Gluten-Free has the flexibility and variety you need to stay on plan, whether you're at the local diner or the best bistro in town. While people with celiac disease, wheat allergy, or gluten sensitivity will need to be on their game when it comes to what they order and how it's prepared, a few basic guidelines can simplify the process.

Do some restaurant research. Before you go out, go online to look at restaurant menus and find meals that follow the guidelines we've set out in this book. Better yet, use the Internet to find local restaurants that accommodate their gluten-free patrons. (It might be easier than you think—there are entire Web sites devoted to cataloging gluten-free hot spots! We have listed a few in our Resources on page 299.)

Plan ahead for special events. If you are attending a party at someone's home and are unsure of the menu, prepare and bring a dish to share that you know you can eat. If the party is at a restaurant or hotel, call the chef or food service manager for information about the menu. Ask if there is a gluten-free menu or whether you can request a special meal. You'll have more success if you call several days to a week in advance. Once you arrive at the party, confirm that your special meal is being prepared and let the kitchen staff know where you are seated.

Get assertive and proactive. Even small traces of gluten will cause cross-contamination—such as bread crumbs that accidentally come in contact with gluten-free food prepared on the same surface or with the same utensils. Be sure to tell the server or chef that it's important to use extra care in preparing and serving your food.

If you get a salad with croutons, send it back and ask for a fresh-made salad to avoid getting the same salad with the croutons picked off. If you don't trust the chef, restaurant, or party host or hostess to deliver a safe, gluten-free meal, eat something at home beforehand and order a beverage, fruit plate, or another safe alternative.

Rely on a safe bet. You can always order a salad of leafy greens and raw veggies, topped with pan-grilled chicken or salmon, and drizzled with olive oil and balsamic vinegar. Add a fist-size serving of one of the following: baked or roasted red, white, or sweet potato; brown or wild rice or a starchy veggie such as beans, peas, or corn. This meal should keep you within your calorie budget and contains a MUFA. Or follow the guidelines for building your own Flat Belly Diet Gluten-Free meal (see Chapter 1).

SATISFYING LEAN PROTEINS

Since one of the goals of Flat Belly Diet Gluten-Free is to reduce the amount of saturated fat you eat, we recommend lean protein, such as skinless poultry, beans, and lean and well-trimmed cuts of beef and pork. (And eat your fish, too!) Here's what lean protein has to offer:

A weight loss advantage. The more muscle you have, the more calories your body burns around the clock. Losing muscle, in contrast, slows your metabolism. Protein contains the amino acid leucine, which helps preserve more muscle while you diet. In a recent study of 48 overweight women dieters, those who ate more protein lost 20 percent more weight than those on an equal-calorie, higher-carb plan, and most of their loss was body fat, not muscle.

Fiber—in meatless protein. You'll enjoy beans several times a week on our plan; they're a good source of soluble fiber, the type that helps control blood sugar. And some varieties, like navy beans and lentils, are also packed with a type of fiber called resistant starch. Because it breaks down extremely slowly in your digestive system, it slows the absorption of sugar into your bloodstream, keeping you fuller longer and protecting you from the physical and emotional ups and downs of a blood sugar spike.

Healthier blood sugar levels. Researchers at the University of Minnesota tested two diets, one high in protein and one with only half as much. The fat content was the same in both diets. In the group that followed the high-protein diet (which was also lower in carbs) for 5 weeks, A1c levels—a test of long-term blood-sugar control—fell by nearly 1 full point, a significant improvement.

FRUITS AND VEGETABLES

This plan's five to eight servings of fruits and vegetables a day are critical for flattening your belly, losing weight, and controlling your blood sugar. Here's why:

They chill systemwide inflammation. Low-level inflammation interferes with the absorption of blood sugar by scrambling signals meant to tell cells to carry sugar molecules inside. But produce cools off inflammation. In a Harvard School of Public Health study of 486 women, those who ate the most produce had the lowest levels of C-reactive protein, a marker of chronic inflammation. Those who ate the most fruit were 34 percent less likely to have metabolic syndrome; those who ate the most veggies cut risk by 30 percent.

They're fiber-full. Fiber fills you up, slows digestion, and slows the release of glucose into your bloodstream. For the most part, fruits and veggies have a low *glycemic load*, a term that refers to how fast and how high carbs boost blood sugar. Including produce at every meal helps slow the rise in your blood sugar afterward. (So do the fats you eat and protein.)

They safeguard your heart. A diet full of fruits and vegetables cuts the risk of heart disease by 28 percent and stroke by 20 percent. One reason: Many fruits and veggies are rich in pectin, a type of water-soluble fiber that helps lower levels of "bad" LDL cholesterol.

A Flatter Belly and Better Health to Boot

We hope you're convinced that you'll enjoy plenty of heart-satisfying food on the Flat Belly Diet! Gluten-Free plan. (And we really hope you dig into the grains listed on page 36. Their flavor can't be beat and they are far more nutritious than plain old white rice.) Moreover, feel free to make those reservations—you'll find plenty to keep you satisfied and on-plan at virtually any eatery (we've listed some sites to find gluten-free dining options in our Resources section on page 299).

Our point: All diets that rein in calories can lead to weight loss, but not all diets can do so deliciously and in ways that actually benefit your health. Flat Belly Diet Gluten-Free goes beyond weight loss. It actually targets belly fat, which is

THE FLAT BELLY DIET GLUTEN-FREE "NO" LIST

If you have been diagnosed with celiac disease or another gluten-related health condition, it's essential that you completely eliminate the foods below. As you can see, the lion's share is wheat and its many varieties of flour.

Keep in mind that wheat is the primary source of gluten in our diets, and that includes many processed foods. For a comprehensive list of foods you need to look at twice, see "Sneaky Sources of Gluten" on page 60.

Wheat	Wheat bran
Spelt	Wheat starch
Einkorn	Wheat germ (only trace amounts are safe)
Emmer	
Kamut	Barley
Durham	Barley malt/Barley extract
Triticale	Brewer's yeast
Bulgur	Rye
Semolina	Oats (unless labeled "gluten free")
Couscous	
Faro	

strongly implicated in inflammatory processes associated with just about every chronic disease.

If you're a gluten-free veteran, you're bound to find Flat Belly Diet Gluten-Free one of the most delicious, satisfying, and effective weight loss plans you've ever tried. If you're a gluten-free newbie, add "easy" to that list of adjectives. We've tried to make gluten-free eating as simple as it is tasty and healthful. Stick to the plan, and you're on your way to a slimmer waistline, healthier blood sugar and cholesterol numbers, boundless energy, and a brighter mood. What you gain is even more important than what you lose. As you shed belly fat, you bolster your health and vitality. Within a few weeks, you'll look slimmer and feel better—all with three mouthwatering meals and two yummy snacks a day!

Of course, maybe you just want to flatten your belly so you're happy with what you see in the mirror. Fine with us! But you'll be healthier, too—and that makes us happy. In the next chapter, you'll take the science behind gluten-free and Flat Belly Diet eating and apply it in the place where all of the plan's benefits begin: your kitchen.

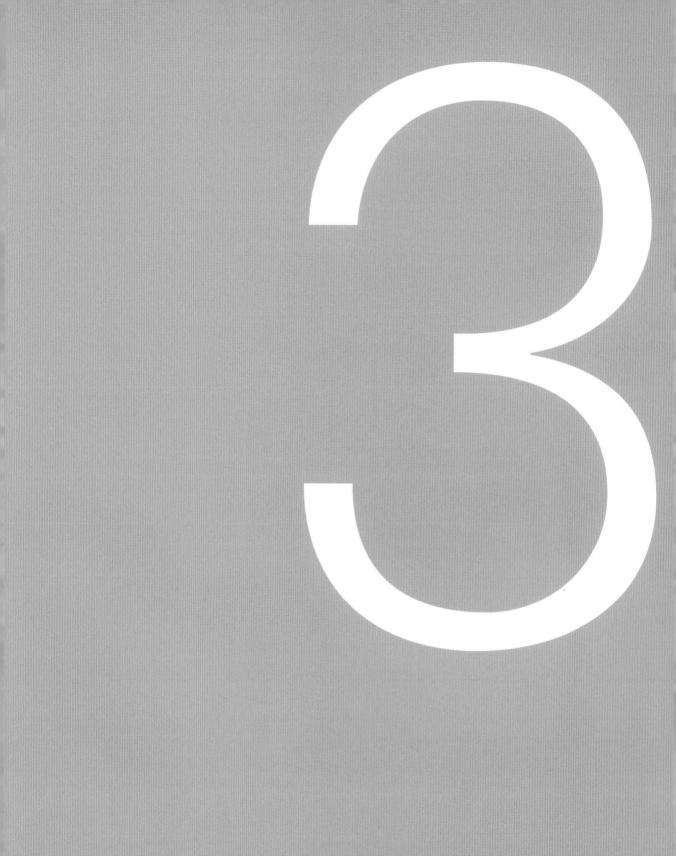

GETTING A FLAT BELLY IN YOUR GLUTEN-FREE KITCHEN

Get ready to shrink your belly as you enjoy tasty, gluten-free meals. On the Flat Belly Diet Gluten-Free plan, success has its own recipe: equal measures of planning and know-how. You'll find that recipe in this chapter.

Start with smart strategies that can help maximize your weight loss while you're on the plan as well as help you sail through those iffy moments that can make or break any dieter. Add a helpful guide to buying, storing, and using MUFAs as well as tips to pump up their flavor. (When you choose quality MUFAs, which are the core of our naturally flavorful way to eat and drop pounds, you're halfway there!)

If you're a gluten-free newbie, no worries. Our pantry guide will help you stock your gluten-free kitchen with all the foods you need to serve up the tasty recipes in this cookbook. (Photocopy the list and take it to the supermarket with you!) And if you're a part-time or full-time vegetarian, you'll learn how to get all the nutrients you need—without the gluten.

When you follow a gluten-free, high-MUFA diet, the trick is to embrace new (and yummy!) foods and find your inner chef. Our guide to gluten-free grains will introduce you to some delicious alternatives to wheat, barley, and rye (such as quinoa, buckwheat, and wild rice), and our quick-and-easy cooking and baking techniques will have you whipping up dazzling MUFA-rich, gluten-free dishes in no time.

Finally, you'll find a selection of deliciously simple recipes for flavored oils, nut toppings, and seasoning mixes that will make any meal mouthwatering. All are gluten and additive free. Think of them as your quick-fix flavorings—though they take just minutes to prepare, you'll use them time and again.

Success in the Kitchen Begins in Your Head

Because our plan centers on foods found to slim your belly, satisfy your hunger, *and* please your tastebuds, it's easy to stick to. But to increase your chances of success, incorporate these simple strategies into your plan from the get-go. They'll keep you focused, feed your motivation, and help you reach your weight loss goal.

STRATEGY #1: EACH NIGHT, PLAN TOMORROW'S MENU

Pick a time of quiet, perhaps each night while you watch TV, to picture where you'll be for each meal and snack. Starting with breakfast, work your way through the next day (sticking, of course, to the rule to eat every 4 hours), and decide now what you'll eat.

Early appointment in the morning? Pack a portable breakfast like Grab-and-Go Breakfast Cups (page 77) before you turn in, and you won't fly out the door hungry and empty-handed. Will your kid's afternoon game interfere with your 4-hours-post-lunchtime snack? Bring along some Peanut Caramel Popcorn (page 247) to munch on while you're cheering, and you won't have to stop for a bag of chips at the minimart or overeat when you finally sit down to dinner. Dining out with friends tomorrow night? Log on to the restaurant's menu online and plan your order in advance. (For more tips, see "Dining Out, Flat Belly Style" on page 37.)

Anticipate potential challenges and plan (and pack food!) to meet them. That way, you'll never be stranded for good options, and you will always avoid missteps that can derail your good intentions.

STRATEGY #2: SCHEDULE IRONCLAD "CART TIME"

If you typically shoehorn your grocery shopping into your day, so that it ranks second or third on your to-do list, here's the hard truth: If you don't have the proper food on hand, it will never find its way into your mouth. So from now on, make shopping a must-do. That way, you'll always have ample supplies on hand for fresh, tasty meals.

In Strategy #1, you're planning what you'll eat tomorrow. Take it a step further and map out which recipes you'd like to try in the coming week.

Once you have a list in hand, decide what shopping time works best for you. If you would rather skip the crowds, avoid hitting the supermarket right after work or at the end of the week or month, when many people get their paychecks. To make it even easier on yourself, pick the same time every week to do your shopping and put that "appointment" on your schedule (if you use a digital calendar, be sure to set a reminder alarm).

Once you upgrade grocery shopping to a must-do on your schedule, treat it like a doctor's appointment you must keep; after all, it's no less important to your health! And every time you keep that commitment, you're showing yourself that your health and well-being count every bit as much as your family's.

STRATEGY #3: MEASURE MORE TO WEIGH LESS

We're not talking about your waist size (although that will shrink soon enough), but about the amounts of ingredients you use as you prepare your meals. Even if you're used to throwing together delicious dishes with a dash of this and a splash of that, measuring your ingredients helps ensure that the Flat Belly Diet Gluten-Free plan controls your hunger and gives you the health and weight loss results you want. Measuring also keeps you mindful of how much you're eating.

Research shows that most people underestimate serving sizes when they eyeball them. Guesstimating measures of MUFAs and other calorie-dense foods is an especially big gamble. For example, say you're unknowingly drizzling 2 tablespoons of olive oil onto your salad instead of the proper MUFA allowance of 1 tablespoon. At 119 calories per tablespoon, making such a miscalculation over and over could seriously hinder your progress.

But the opposite is also true: If you don't measure out your 2 delicious tablespoons of peanut butter, you may not get every last bit that's coming to you. Even if 2 tablespoons seems like a lot to you, resist any urge to use less. If you reduce the amount, not only will you take in less MUFA overall, but your hunger might return more quickly and throw off your meal timing. So measure away and enjoy!

STRATEGY #4: LEARN TO SOOTHE A HUNGRY HEART

You finished your snack half an hour ago when, out of nowhere, you're blindsided by a massive craving for ice cream. Rather than agonize over whether to hit the drive-thru, ask these two questions:

○ Has this hunger come on suddenly?

○ Am I craving a specific food or type of food?

Sudden onset is a telltale sign of emotional hunger. True physical hunger, on the other hand, comes on gradually. And a craving for a specific food (such as that ice cream) or a type of food (something salty) is another clear sign of emotional hunger. When you learn to spot hunger pangs that radiate from above the neck, it will get easier to tune them out and listen to your belly instead. (If it's rumbling, your body needs food.)

Once you've determined that your hunger is emotional rather than physical, head for the nearest full-length mirror. Take stock of the visible results you've achieved thus far. They're tangible proof that what you are doing is right for you. It took a leap of faith—in yourself—to get you here. Honor your commitment to yourself and go the distance. You deserve success.

STRATEGY #5: CELEBRATE THE LEANER, HEALTHIER YOU

It never fails. You're in the zone, doing great, and then *bam*—an office birthday party, a holiday family dinner, or drinks with friends. Suddenly, you're on shaky ground. Everyone is eating—cheese puffs, birthday cake, Mom's signature lasagna (gluten, gluten everywhere!), and it's hard to just say no.

Whether it's pressure to "just have a little" from family and friends, a waiter who betrays his impatience with your questions about a particular dish, or a hostess who's "hurt" that you haven't sampled her famous crab dip, social situations can be tough. It's especially hard if you feel deprived and turn your focus on the foods you're giving up.

When that happens, shift your focus. Take a moment to reflect on what you're getting. A slimmer figure. A longer, healthier life. A new attitude about food—that it's a pleasure, rather than a source of guilt and fear. An opportunity to motivate others, perhaps people you love, to change their lifestyles and their lives. The fun of bringing a healthy dish from this cookbook to your next social engagement or family dinner, and not telling them it's healthy until after they've exclaimed how delicious it is.

That's a lot of perks to focus on! So the next time a social situation makes you second-guess your resolve, take a moment to remember them. Chances are, you'll feel a new confidence in the choices you've made, and they'll taste better than anything on the buffet table.

MUFA-licious! How to Buy and Use the Flat Belly Foods

Nutritious, versatile, and easy to use, MUFA foods are some of the most delicious on planet Earth. However, it's important to buy the best you can afford, store them properly, and use them in ways that maximize both their flavor and their nutritional benefits.

With every tasty bite, the foods on this plan work hard to fight belly fat, help you lose extra pounds, and more. Here's what you need to know.

OILS

Buy them: Choose oils based on how you'll use them (cooking or drizzling) and on flavor (strong or mild). Look for oils that are expeller-pressed, a chemical-free extraction process that lets the oil keep its natural color, aroma, and nutrients. Delicate oils like flaxseed should be cold-pressed, which means they're pressed in temperatures below 120 degrees. Only buy an amount you'll use in about 2 months. Any longer than that, and the oil will deteriorate and become stale and bitter.

Store them: Keep most oils in a cool, dark place, like the back of your pantry. Exceptions: Flaxseed and walnut oils do best in the refrigerator; they break down more quickly in warm temperatures.

Use them: Drizzle oil on salads, veggies, and grilled meats and fish, or into marinades and dressings. Pick up an oil "mister" at a kitchen gadget store. It allows you to spray a fine mist of oil on foods.

Tip: Use dark glass jars or tins (rather than clear plastic or glass bottles) to protect those precious oils from light, a source of flavor-sapping oxidation.

Most MUFA for the money: Safflower oil labeled "high oleic" contains the most MUFAs, followed by olive and canola oils.

Serving: 1 tablespoon

OLIVES AND TAPENADE

Buy them: Besides jarred or canned olives, you'll find a great selection—black or green, salty, sweet or spicy—at many grocery store deli counters or olive bars. They may also be flavored with herbs or hot chiles. For a change of pace from the fruit itself, pick up a jarred tapenade that lists olives as the main ingredient and contains about 40 calories per tablespoon. As always, read the ingredients list carefully.

Store them: Keep olives and tapenade in their original jars or in airtight containers in the refrigerator. If you buy olives in cans, transfer any left over into an airtight container and store them in the fridge.

Use them: Yummy by themselves as a snack or appetizer, olives can also be tossed into salads or included in meat dishes and pasta sauce. Though olives and tapenades are rich in healthy fats, they also tend to be salty, so limit olive dishes to one per day to keep your sodium intake in check.

Tip: The next time you fix a sandwich, spread on a serving of tapenade. It's a delicious alternative to traditional condiments like ketchup and mayonnaise.

Most MUFA for the money: Pop the olives you enjoy! All varieties provide almost three-quarters of their fat as oleic acid.

Serving: 10 olives or 2 tablespoons tapenade

TASTY TAPENADE

When you're looking for a little something to spread on your gluten-free bread or crackers, turn to tapenade. In the regional cuisine of Provence, France, this thick, delicious paste made from black olives, capers, anchovies, and olive oil is a traditional condiment. It may also include lemon juice, basil or other herbs, liqueur such as brandy, mustard, and sometimes bits of tuna.

Here in the United States, food manufacturers use the word *tapenade* to advertise spreads or dips made from "Mediterranean" ingredients. This means that the tapenades in the deli case or condiments aisle may contain green olives rather than the traditional black—or no olives at all, much less the other traditional ingredients. Some ready-made tapenades contain artichokes, sun-dried tomatoes, roasted red peppers, or even figs.

To count as a MUFA, a packaged tapenade must list olives as a main ingredient. The tapenade you buy should also be labeled "gluten free." If it's not, check the ingredients carefully to ensure they do not include gluten-containing fillers or additives. Keep an eye on the nutrition label, too: Each tablespoon should contain about 40 calories.

We suggest that you make your own tapenade. It's easy, gives you control over the ingredients, and is sure to yield a spread that better pleases your palate. You can adjust the proportions of the basic ingredients to your liking and experiment with additional ingredients—a dash of lemon juice here, a pinch of oregano there. Plus, you save money. Store-bought tapenades can be pricey! You'll find our yummy gluten-free recipe on page 80.

NUTS, NUT BUTTERS, AND SEEDS

Buy them: Select nuts that are labeled "plain" and/or "raw." Avoid oil-roasted or salted varieties, which add extra fat and calories as well as sodium (dry-roasted without salt are fine). Bypass nuts that are dark, mottled, or shriveled. Never buy nuts in their shells from a bulk bin, to avoid cross-contamination with gluten. Bypass additive-packed nut butters and look for brands labeled "all natural." Your pick should contain only small amounts of salt, oil, or sugar (which may be listed as molasses or evaporated cane juice). Steer clear of seeds that are discolored or shriveled or smell rancid or musty.

Store them: Stash nuts and seeds in airtight containers and keep them in a cool, dry place like your pantry. Raw, unshelled nuts will last 6 to 12 months; shelled nuts keep 3 to 4 months. You can also freeze shelled nuts for up to a year. Natural nut butters have a layer of oil on top, and trying to mix it is a sloppy task. So store the jar upside down to incorporate the oil back into the nut butter and keep opened jars in the refrigerator. If you find it hard to spread, remove the lid and warm the jar in the microwave for 10 seconds, or spoon your serving into a glass dish and heat.

Use them: Sprinkle nuts and seeds onto salads and cooked veggies, or into gluten-free pasta, yogurt, gluten-free cereal, or gluten-free pancake or muffin batter. Chop or grind them up for a crunchy coating for fish or chicken. Or toss them with dried fruit in a resealable plastic bag for an easy, on-the-go snack. Swirl a gluten-free nut butter, such as Smart Balance Peanut Butter, into gluten-free oatmeal, blend it into smoothies, or spread it onto gluten-free waffles or crackers. It's tasty on apple slices, too.

Tip: Store nuts in mason jars on your kitchen counter, away from direct sunlight, to keep these frequently used ingredients stylishly accessible.

Most MUFA for the money: Macadamia nuts provide more MUFAs than any other nut or seed.

Serving: 2 tablespoons

SURPRISE: EAT NUTS, WEIGH LESS

Although they're high in fat, eating nuts does not lead to weight gain. In fact, research suggests that they may help people manage their weight better. For instance, in a 2007 Spanish study of 8,865 people, those who ate nuts at least twice a week were less likely to gain weight over a more than 2-year period than those who never or rarely ate them.

Even when people add nuts to their usual diets, they don't seem to gain. In a small 2007 study from Purdue University, women added 344 calories worth of almonds a day to their diets and neither ate less nor exercised more. After 10 weeks, they hadn't gained weight. But there's nothing magical about almonds keeping off weight. Studies on walnuts and peanuts have reported similar findings.

The bottom line, according to a 2007 scientific review of nuts and body weight: When added freely to a diet, nuts cause less weight gain than would be predicted, and when added to a calorie-controlled diet, they don't cause weight gain and may make weight loss easier.

How can indulging in such a fat-rich treat help you avoid packing on pounds? Researchers think that the fiber and protein in nuts help make you feel full longer, so you're less hungry and eat less at your next meal. And there's some evidence that nuts may affect metabolism in a way that compensates for the high calories they contain.

AVOCADOS

Buy them: Select fruits that are firm or give just slightly when gently pressed. Bypass those that are bruised, cracked, or indented. Scan ingredient lists on guacamole. Avocado should be listed first.

Store them: To ripen a very hard avocado, keep it on the counter for 24 to 48 hours; putting it into a paper bag will shorten ripening by a day. Keep ripe avocados in the refrigerator and use within 1 or 2 days.

Use them: Avocados can be mashed for dips or spreads, or sliced and chopped for sandwiches or salads.

Tip: To prevent a leftover portion of avocado from turning brown, coat the exposed flesh with lemon juice, wrap tightly in plastic wrap, and store in the refrigerator.

Most MUFA for the money: Compared to avocados from Florida, Hass avocados provide almost twice the amount of MUFAs per ¼-cup serving.

Serving: One-fourth of an avocado (about ¼ cup)

HOW TO PIT AND PEEL AN AVOCADO

To pit an avocado, use a small serrated knife to cut through the skin and around the pit lengthwise. Twist the halves apart. If the pit remains attached, gently press the serrated knife into the pit until the blade bites into it and then lift the pit from the flesh. To remove the pit from the knife, tap it on the edge of a sink or trash can.

To peel an avocado, place the halves cut side down. Cut 2 equally spaced lengthwise slits just through the skin. With the edge of a knife blade, lift the top corner of each strip and peel back the skin. Or scoop the avocado out of the peel with a spoon.

DARK CHOCOLATE

Buy it: Check labels for the words *semisweet*, *bittersweet*, or *extra bittersweet*. Choose chocolate that contains at least 60 percent cacao. Stock up on chips, bars, and chunks. (Many of Hershey's chocolate chunks and chips are gluten free, but always check the label before you buy.)

Store it: Keep unopened chocolate in a cool, dry place (not above 75°F or you risk a soft, gooey mess). Opened chocolate should be stored in an airtight container or bag in the refrigerator or freezer. Stored chocolate may develop a slightly white coating, which is perfectly safe to eat.

Use it: Savor it straight up, melted onto fresh fruit, baked into gluten-free muffins or quick breads, grated into gluten-free oatmeal or yogurt—we're sure you will think of something!

Tip: If you're used to milk chocolate, go dark gradually—from semisweet (you've eaten it in cookies!) to extra bittersweet—so you train your tastebuds to appreciate the stronger, richer flavor of real chocolate.

Most MUFA for the money: Because all dark chocolate contains rich amounts of MUFAs, select your favorite. Never tasted dark chocolate? To get the scoop on our dark chocolate taste test, see the chart below.

Serving: 1 ounce or ¼ cup chips

Dark Chocolate Brands Compared Side by Side

Each of these brands is certified gluten free as of this printing, but be sure to check labels each time you buy.

	ENDANGERED SPECIES CHOCOLATE COMPANY: DARK CHOCOLATE WITH DEEP FOREST MINT	DOVE: RICH DARK CHOCOLATE	ITHACA FINE CHOCOLATES: ART BAR EXQUISITE SWISS DARK CHOCOLATE WITH COCONUT	SCHARFFEN BERGER CHOCOLATE MAKER: 70% CACAO BITTERSWEET CHOCOLATE BAR	DAGOBA: ROSEBERRY DARK CHOCOLATE BAR
Description	70% cocoa; 10% of profits are donated to protecting endangered animals	Made with Cocoapro (specially processed cocoa designed to preserve high levels of heart-healthy flavonoids); individually wrapped squares	Minimum 58% cocoa with coconut; certified organic Swiss chocolate; Fair Trade certified; 10% of profits go to art education programs	70% cocoa	59% cocoa blended with dried raspberries and bits of rose hips; 100% organic; supports Fair Trade
Comments	"This one turned me into a dark chocolate lover," said one tester. Staffers loved the balance of mint and cocoa and the charitable tie-in.	"Like velvet," remarked a taster. Dove was a unanimous fave among editors.	"Like a chocolate-dipped macaroon," one muncher said. Coconut shavings added great texture.	Staffers tested a variety of bars from this brand, but the bittersweet was juuust right for its smooth, melt-in-your-mouth flavor.	"Loved the tart, sweet bits of raspberry blended into a decadent dark chocolate," commented a choco-maniac.
Nutritional Lowdown	Serving size: ½ bar (1.5 oz); 250 cal, 2 g pro, 23 g carb, 16 g fat, 10 g sat fat, 0 mg chol, 3 g fiber, 50 mg sodium, 17 g sugar	Serving size: 5 pieces (1.4 oz); 210 cal, 2 g pro, 24 g carb, 13 g fat, 8 g sat fat, 5 mg chol, 3 g fiber, 0 mg sodium, 19 g sugar	Serving size: about ⅓ bar (1.4 oz); 200 cal, 2 g pro, 21 g carb, 15 g fat, 10 g sat fat, 0 mg chol, 6 g fiber, 0 mg sodium, 13 g sugar	Serving size: ½ bar (1.5 oz); 250 cal, 3 g pro, 20 g carb, 18 g fat, 11 g sat fat, 0 mg chol, <1 g fiber, 0 mg sodium, 13 g sugar	Serving size: ½ bar (1 oz); 157 cal, 1 g pro,17 g carb, 9 g fat, 6 g sat fat, 0 mg chol, 3 g fiber, 0 mg sodium, 12 g sugar
Cost and Where to Buy	$2.75 per bar; natural food stores; www.chocolatebar.com	$3 per bag; grocery stores (United States only)	$3 per bar; www.ithacafinechocolates.com	$4.25 per bar; www.scharffenberger.com (United States only)	$2.89 per bar; natural food stores; www.dagobachocolate.com

Stocking Your Flat Belly Diet Gluten-Free Pantry

We at *Prevention* are label mavens: We always want to know what's in our food and how much of it. When you shop for a gluten-free diet, it's doubly important to read food labels—every food, every time you shop. While all the staples on our pantry list are "Go" foods, any packaged food should be labeled "gluten free" before it goes in your cart. These guidelines can help make sure you buy right.

Watch for these words. If a food is not labeled "gluten free," read the ingredients list and the "Contains" statement on the label. In general, any of these words means the food contains gluten: *wheat, barley, rye, malt* (unless a gluten-free source is named, like *corn malt*), *brewer's yeast*, and *oats* (only oats labeled "gluten free" are safe to eat). Also, unless a gluten-free grain is named as the source, avoid foods with these words: *malt, malt flavoring*, and *modified food starch*. Modified food starch can be safe, however, if the "Contains" statement doesn't include wheat.

Be particular about dairy. The Flat Belly Diet Gluten-Free plan recommends fat-free and low-fat dairy products, which typically contain fillers or other ingredients that contain gluten. Buy only those dairy products labeled "gluten free."

Be aware that gluten is everywhere. It's in soy sauce, nondairy coffee creamer, and countless other packaged foods, so be sure to read "Sneaky Sources of Gluten" on page 60. (Foods that people with celiac disease should absolutely avoid—called "No" foods—are listed in Chapter 2.)

Gluten-free shopping has a learning curve, but keep your eyes on the prize: better health and a slimmer belly. You'll get the hang of it sooner than you think!

GRAINS FOR THE GLUTEN-FREE GOURMET

While the names of these grains may sound strange, they're 100 percent delicious. To sample them, go on a grains safari, either in the organic food section of your local supermarket or a local natural foods store. You can enjoy them in dozens of ways—as a sweet hot cereal or savory side dish, in soups and stews, and as flour for pancakes, muffins, and quick breads. They're usually made into cold, ready-to-eat cereal, too.

Amaranth: A sacred food to the ancient Aztecs, this grain has a cornlike

THE GLUTEN-FREE VEGETARIAN

Yes, you can follow a vegetarian diet and still lose weight on the Flat Belly Diet Gluten-Free plan. (Every one of those delicious MUFAs is naturally gluten free!) To ensure that you get all the nutrients your body needs as you outsmart sneaky sources of gluten, keep a few things in mind.

Read your labels. Many foods that are mainstays of the vegetarian diet contain, or may contain, gluten. These include grain- or nut-based milks, meat alternatives, and Asian products like seasoned tofu or tempeh, miso, seitan, and tamari sauce. As always, CTL—Check the Label.

Mind your vitamins and minerals. On the Flat Belly Diet Gluten-Free plan, you'll eat plenty of nutrient-rich fruits, veggies, and nongluten grains. However, when you're a gluten-free vegetarian, it's more of a challenge to get adequate amounts of vitamins B_{12} and D and the minerals calcium, zinc, and iron. And you can't depend on gluten-free breakfast cereals—most aren't fortified. Fortunately, there are plenty of gluten-free vegetarian sources of these must-have nutrients:

O **Vitamin B_{12}:** eggs, Cheddar cheese, low-fat yogurt, and specific brands of nut- or grain-based milks (Silk Soy or Rice Dream)

O **Vitamin D:** eggs, gluten-free Rice Chex (General Mills), specific brands of orange juice (Minute Maid Calcium + D, Tropicana Calcium + D), specific brands of nut- or grain-based "milks" (Silk Soy, Rice Dream, Pacific Natural Foods)

O **Calcium:** cooked greens (kale, spinach, turnip, beet, or mustard greens), calcium-fortified orange juice, stewed tomatoes

O **Zinc:** Cheddar cheese, low-fat yogurt, most kinds of beans, quinoa, walnuts, and almonds. Soaking dried beans before you cook them may increase the availability of zinc.

O **Iron:** seeds (pumpkin, flax, sesame, sunflower), quinoa, amaranth, gluten-free oats, teff, sorghum, millet, soybeans, pulses, almonds, peanuts, dried apricots, prunes and raisins, cooked spinach, baked potato (with the skin), green peas, acorn squash, Brussels sprouts, blackstrap molasses, enriched gluten-free bread products, cereals, and pasta

Mind your protein. Gluten-free soy-based meat alternatives are hard to find, so it's important to eat a wide variety of plant protein throughout the day so you get an adequate intake of indispensable amino acids. Grains that don't contain gluten, including quinoa and brown rice, and many varieties of beans, lentils, split peas, nuts and seeds, and tofu are good sources of protein.

aroma and woodsy flavor. For a hearty main dish, mix it with beans. Cook it in fruit juice or water, and add a small amount of chopped fruit and nuts, and it becomes a delicious hot breakfast cereal.

Buckwheat: Buckwheat's hard outer hull contains a kernel called the groat. Whole groats are cooked as a side dish or added to soups, stuffings, stews, and casseroles. Ground groats are cooked as a hot cereal or made into flour mixed with varying amounts of the crushed hulls. Dark buckwheat flour, which contains more hulls, has a stronger, more distinctive flavor than the lighter flour.

Millet: The most common variety in North America is light yellow millet and has a slight cornlike, sweet, nutty flavor. It can be cooked in water or broth and eaten alone as a cereal, as a side dish such as pilaf, or used for poultry stuffing or as a salad. Puffed millet is excellent as a cold cereal or—when crushed—as breading.

Quinoa: A native South American grain with a soft, crunchy texture, quinoa boasts the highest nutritional profile of all grains—it's often called a supergrain. It contains more high-quality protein than other grains and cereals.

Sorghum: Use this small, round seed, slightly larger than a peppercorn, in pilaf; add to casseroles, stuffings, or salads; or use as an alternative to rice in pudding. Ground into flour, sorghum's mild flavor won't compete with the flavors of other ingredients.

Teff: This tiny cereal grain—about 100 to 150 teff grains equal the size of one wheat kernel—has a nutty, mild, molasses-like flavor. You can eat it as a hot cereal, in a side dish or casseroles, or cold in salads. You can also find pasta made from teff.

Wild rice: You can enjoy its chewy texture and nutty, roasted flavor alone or use it in casseroles, salads, or side dishes.

Now that you know which grains are gluten free, here are a few ways to enjoy them.

- Enjoy hot cereal for breakfast—gluten-free oats, buckwheat flakes, hot quinoa.

- Sprinkle cooked whole grains over salads.

- Toss cooked whole grains with gluten-free pasta.

- For a taste of the Southwest, blend brown rice with black or pinto beans.

- Toss cold cooked whole grains with a zesty gluten-free salad dressing.

WHAT IS CROSS-CONTAMINATION?

Whether you're a gluten-free expert or just trying this eating style for the first time, it's crucial to know the facts about cross-contamination—the unintentional contact of a gluten-free food with wheat, barley, or rye. Cross-contamination has the potential to happen any time a gluten-free food comes into contact with wheat, barley, or rye. Eating cross-contaminated foods can be a danger to you if you have celiac disease or a gluten sensitivity because you risk exposure to gluten from unsuspected sources.

It's important to know that cross-contamination can happen at any stage in the process of making, packaging, or transporting gluten-free foods. For example, gluten-free grains might journey in railcars or trucks that have previously held wheat, barley, or rye. Or manufacturing plants might have made gluten-free products on the same lines as foods that contain gluten. Cross-contamination can even occur in your own kitchen—for example, if you prepare gluten-free foods with a cutting board, microwave tray, or colander that has come into contact with gluten. (See "Avoid Cross-Contamination in the Kitchen" on page 63).

It sounds scary, but manufacturers of gluten-free products are keenly aware of the potential for cross-contamination and take stringent measures to avoid it. They may make gluten-free foods on separate production lines or even in separate facilities dedicated solely to gluten-free products. There are other safeguards, too. Most manufacturers test their raw ingredients *and* finished products for gluten and periodically have independent labs test their gluten-free products for the presence of gluten.

GO FOR PURE OATS

Oats are one of the healthiest foods you can eat, brimming with protein, fiber, iron, and B vitamins. But it's also true that some packaged oats and oat products can be cross-contaminated with wheat, rye, and/or barley. Fortunately, there are companies that produce uncontaminated oats, grown on dedicated fields and processed in dedicated gluten-free facilities. These specialty gluten-free oat companies include:

- Cream Hill Estates
- Gifts of Nature

○ GF Harvest (formerly Gluten Free Oats)

○ Only Oats from Avena

○ PrOatina

○ Bob's Red Mill

While most people with celiac disease can eat moderate amounts of pure, uncontaminated oats, a small number may not. Individuals with celiac disease should always check in with their doctor or dietitian before adding them to their gluten-free diet.

SWEETS

You shouldn't need any store-bought sweets or desserts—we've got plenty of delectable gluten-free treats beginning on page 257. Keep in mind that it is difficult to find gluten-free sweets that are fat free or low calorie, and that these types of products tend to contain a lot of fat.

When it comes to making your own desserts or just having sweeteners on hand, our top choices are listed on page 58. Use low-calorie versions, if you can find them, but check labels for added ingredients that may not be gluten free. If you can't find low-calorie, gluten-free substitutes, use these sweeteners sparingly or not at all.

CONDIMENTS

Dressings and other condiments used on the Flat Belly Diet Gluten-Free plan should be fat free and/or low calorie as well as gluten free. For a list of suggested sauces to have in your pantry, check out our list on page 59.

BEVERAGES

Many drinks are safe for consumption on a gluten-free diet. Most teas, coffees, hot chocolate mixes, and ciders are safe (for a full list, see page 59). And although you shouldn't be drinking them *regularly* as part of the Flat Belly Diet, the following are generally gluten free: soft drinks, pure distilled alcoholic beverages (i.e., rum, whiskey, vodka), wine (red and white), and most liqueurs.

YOUR PANTRY CHECKLIST

DAIRY PRODUCTS

- ○ Egg whites (or cholesterol-reduced liquid egg product)
- ○ Plain soy milk or fat-free milk
- ○ Fat-free vanilla yogurt
- ○ Fat-free sour cream
- ○ Aged cheeses (i.e., Cheddar, Swiss, Edam, Parmesan)
- ○ Blue cheese
- ○ Most processed cheese
- ○ Fat-free cottage cheese
- ○ Fat-free cream cheese or soft cheeses

GRAIN PRODUCTS*

- ○ Amaranth
- ○ Arrowroot
- ○ Buckwheat
- ○ Cassava, manioc, tapioca, yucca (starches ground from the roots of these individual plants)
- ○ Chia seed
- ○ Corn
- ○ Flaxseed
- ○ Mesquite (flour made from the mesquite tree, a member of the legume family)
- ○ Millet
- ○ Montina
- ○ Oats**
- ○ Quinoa
- ○ Rice
- ○ Sago (a starch from the sago palm plant)
- ○ Sorghum (a round, berrylike, cream-colored grain available in grain and flour form)
- ○ Soy
- ○ Teff
- ○ Wild rice

*Because of cross-contamination concerns, any product made from even these grains should be labeled "gluten free."

**Because oats are often cross-contaminated with wheat, barley, and rye, take special care to select only oats labeled "gluten free."

FRUITS AND VEGETABLES

- ○ All plain fresh, frozen, and canned fruits
- ○ Fruit juices
- ○ All plain fresh, frozen, dried, and canned vegetables
- ○ Pure vegetable juices (such as V8)
- ○ Plain tomato sauce
- ○ Plain tomato paste
- ○ Spaghetti sauce made with allowed ingredients
- ○ Fresh potatoes

MEATS AND OTHER PROTEIN FOODS

- ○ Plain meat, poultry, and fish
- ○ Plain lentils, chickpeas, peas, and beans
- ○ Most peanut butters
- ○ All natural peanut butters
- ○ Plain tofu

FATS

- MUFAs! (Avocados, olives, plain nuts and seeds, all MUFA oils except wheat germ oil)
- Sweets
- Honey
- Maple syrup
- Jelly, jam, marmalade
- Molasses
- Sugar (white and brown)
- Coconut
- Fructose
- Artificial sweeteners
- Pure cocoa powder
- Carob chips and pure carob powder (check ingredients carefully)
- Most chocolate syrups
- Some rice syrups (buy only rice syrup labeled "gluten free")

CONDIMENTS

- Relish
- Ketchup
- Most prepared mustards (some mustards contain wheat)
- Olives
- Most salad dressings
- Most mayonnaise
- Most vinegars except malt vinegar and some flavored vinegars
- Tahini
- Low-sodium soy sauce made without wheat
- All pure spices and herbs, including pure black pepper and mustard flour (Check ingredients of mustard flour to ensure the only ingredient is ground mustard seeds.)
- Salt-free seasonings

BEVERAGES

- Pure tea
- Most herbal teas
- Coffee (instant or ground)
- Pure cocoa powder and most hot chocolate mixes
- Cider
- Some soy beverages

SOUPS AND MISCELLANEOUS

- Homemade soups using gluten-free ingredients; gluten-free bouillon cubes and broth
- Sauces and gravies thickened without flour and made without gluten-based flavorings
- Pure vanilla extract
- Baking soda, yeast (except brewer's yeast), most baking powder, cream of tartar, cornstarch
- Corn gluten, corn malt
- Corn tacos, corn tortillas (labeled "gluten free")
- Miso—plain, rice, or soybean
- Gluten-free pizza crust
- Gums: xanthan, guar, carrageenan, acacia, carob bean, cellulose, arabic, locust bean, tragacanth
- Plain popcorn
- Plain rice cakes
- Plain popped corn cakes

SNEAKY SOURCES OF GLUTEN

Because gluten travels under several assumed names, it's often hard to spot on food labels. If the food is not labeled "gluten free," remember to look for wheat, barley, rye, oats, malt, or brewer's yeast in the ingredients list. Here are a few of the foods that may contain "undercover gluten."

- Bouillon cubes
- Cereal
- Cooking spray
- Dairy substitutes
- Herbal teas (some)
- Ice cream with added mix-ins
- Instant coffee
- Licorice
- Marshmallows
- Meat sauce
- Prepared cake frosting
- Processed cheeses
- Salad dressing
- Sauces and gravies
- Soup (mixes and cans)
- Soy sauce
- Yogurt

In our recipes, we call for a number of ingredients that require careful checking of labels. Some of these products include deli meats, such as sausage and bacon; balsamic vinaigrette; rice vinegar; various mustards; seasoning mixes; polenta; and semisweet chocolate chips. Always read labels carefully to avoid sources of gluten.

Cooking the Flat Belly Gluten-Free Way

MUFA foods are a foodie's dream come true—lovely to look at, full of flavor, satisfying, and healthy to boot. However, because MUFA foods are high in fat, you'll want to cook them in ways that add flavor, not unnecessary fat and calories.

The cooking techniques below are our go-to methods—quick and easy, low in fat and sodium, and well suited to bringing out the full flavor of MUFA foods. We've even provided a few tried-and-true test kitchen tips for each method.

ROASTING: GIVE VEGGIES A FLAVOR MAKEOVER

To transform virtually any veggie from bland to mind-blowing, toss a pan of them with a drizzle of canola oil, a pinch of kosher salt, and freshly ground black pepper. Then roast them at around 400°F until nicely browned (30 to 45 minutes).

The veggies should have crisp edges and tender middles. (Poke them with a fork to test.)

Roast in a shallow baking dish, the bottom of a broiler pan, or a rimmed baking sheet. The hot air surrounds the veggies and browns them nicely. Avoid deep casserole dishes and don't cover the dish, or you won't get the desirable color or crispness.

If you're new to roasting, you're in for a treat! Pale, mild-tasting cauliflower caramelizes to golden brown and takes on a rich, nutty flavor. Brussels sprouts are neither bitter nor mushy, but sweet and pleasingly tender-crisp. Carrots go from run-of-the-mill to savory. Sliced first into thin circles, roasted potatoes have a crispy, chiplike crust surrounding a tender center—for flavor, they rival french fries. To add color, nutrients, and even more flavor, combine roasted potatoes with slivered yams.

SLOW-COOKING: TASTY MEALS FOR THE TIME-PRESSED

Set it and forget it, but when mealtime comes, savor it! Whatever goes into a slow cooker—low-fat proteins, lean cuts of meat, dried beans—slow-cooks to succulent perfection. Slow cookers are indispensable for cooks who want to maximize flavor and minimize fat, and who need a flavorful, healthy meal to be ready the minute they walk in the door.

Slow-cooking has a few basic guidelines. For example, cut raw meat into pieces and place them at the bottom of the slow cooker so that they heat up relatively quickly, and make sure cooking times are specific to your appliance (they're different for a 3-quart versus a 6-quart cooker).

New to slow-cooking? Don't leave those instructions at the bottom of the box. Before you fire up your new slow cooker, read the accompanying manual, especially the directions concerning food safety.

GRILLING: A SWEET TECHNIQUE FOR FLAVORFUL MEAT

Cooking over a flame drains off fat while imparting delicious smoky flavor to meat, chicken, and seafood. Keep grilling simple and speedy: Choose proteins that cook within 25 minutes over direct heat, such as steaks and chops, chicken pieces, fish steaks, tofu, and burgers. Or skewer variations of these in cubed or meatball form.

To keep meat, fish, or poultry moist and flavorful, sear it on all sides to lock in juices, and marinate it (in a gluten-free marinade) before grilling. If you like, baste with a gluten-free marinade a few times while cooking. Cook seafood just until opaque at the center, but don't rely on visual appearance to judge doneness of meat or chicken. Instead, invest in an instant-read thermometer, which is more reliable. Remove meat from the grill when it's within 10 degrees of doneness. Set aside for several minutes while the temperature continues to rise. It's ready to serve when the thermometer reaches the temperature for doneness.

POACHING: PERFECT FOR FISH

To infuse flavor without adding fat, immerse fillets of any mild-flavored, firm-fleshed fish (we like salmon, sea bass, cod, and halibut) in barely simmering liquid and cook until just opaque all the way through—roughly 20 to 30 minutes, depending on thickness. From this supremely simple technique comes intensely savory flavor.

To whip up a simple poaching liquid, chop 2 carrots, a celery stalk, and an onion, and add them to a pan of water with a splash of vinegar or lemon juice. Toss in a few whole peppercorns, a bay leaf, a sprinkling of kosher salt, and any fresh herbs (dill is excellent) you happen to have in the fridge. Remove the fish and veggies when done and turn up the heat to reduce the poaching liquid to a sauce.

STIR-FRYING: TASTY, HEALTHY ONE-DISH MEALS IN MINUTES

A little oil and a lot of heat add up to a superfast low-fat cooking method. Stir-frying requires some slicing and dicing up front, but pays off big with meals that cook up in as little as 10 minutes. Another advantage of stir-frying: It allows you to experiment with unlimited combinations of proteins and vegetables. Thin strips or slices cook quickly and evenly over high heat—vegetables retain flavor and crisp-tenderness, while proteins stay tender.

No time to chop veggies? Buy them prewashed and precut. Or hit the super-market salad bar for a wide variety of ready-to-cook veggies. Here are our favorite stir-fry secrets: Roll tofu cubes or strips of chicken in sesame seeds for a delicious crunch. Use baby vegetables, which are sweet (to look at and to taste) and require little to no prep. Stir in a cup of frozen chopped spinach (slightly thawed) for 1 minute before your stir-fry is done to add color, flavor, and body-nourishing iron.

AVOID CROSS-CONTAMINATION IN THE KITCHEN

If you've been diagnosed with celiac disease, this message is for you: If any portion of your gluten-free meal comes into contact with ingredients that contain gluten, the result could be uncomfortable, even harmful. Remember—even a speck of gluten can ruin your day! So how do you prevent contact, especially when you share a kitchen?

To stay safe and healthy, take care before, during, and after preparing your gluten-free meals—and make sure friends, family, and restaurants follow these guidelines, too.

O In your pantry, freezer, and fridge, store all gluten-free products (including gluten-free breads, crackers, pastas, mixes, and more) apart from foods that contain gluten.

O Buy two jars of anything eaten on gluten-free bread, such as peanut butter, jelly, and mayonnaise—and be sure to label which jar is gluten free and which is for regular bread. If that doesn't work for your family, institute a strict rule: When it comes to foods in jars, absolutely no double-dipping allowed. Once the utensil touches the bread, it doesn't go back into the jar!

O Buy two sets of kitchen tools (cutting boards, colanders, serving spoons, tongs, and so forth). It might help to make the gluten-free tools of a different make or color, or mark them with a bit of bright duct tape. Alternatively, prepare gluten-free foods first, followed by gluten-containing foods, and scrub the tools well after each use.

O If your microwave oven or grill is used to prepare foods that contain gluten, keep these appliances scrupulously clean; wash them or wipe them down with a mild detergent or soap after each use, and then dry them thoroughly.

O When microwaving gluten-free foods, *always* use a clean plate rather than one that has just been used to microwave gluten-containing foods. It's also helpful to have separate splatter covers. (You can mark the gluten-free cover with duct tape.)

O If possible, get a separate toaster oven for gluten-free breads to avoid getting crumbs from regular bread on your slices. Or lay your gluten-free bread on aluminum foil. You might also use toaster bags, available online. If you've never heard of these nifty little items, toaster bags are little plastic pouches that you can tuck your gluten-free bread into. You can use them to heat pizza and make grilled cheese, too! Most can be reused and are dishwasher safe.

Scrumptious Staples: Oils, Mixes, and More

Whether you're whipping up a salad or looking for a quick, MUFA-rich snack, you'll return to these quick-and-easy recipes for flavor-infused oils, flavored nuts, and seasoning mixes time and again. And because you're making them yourself, you know they're gluten free.

INFUSED OILS

There are plenty of great-tasting MUFA-rich oils to choose from, but loading up on all of them at once can get pricey. Instead, use the following recipes to add a twist to your basic olive oil or approximate the flavor of a nut oil. Remember that olive oil becomes cloudy when refrigerated but quickly returns to its clear hue when brought to room temperature.

Garlic-Infused Oil (*makes 2 cups*)

4–6 cloves garlic, thinly sliced

6 large green olives, coarsely chopped

1 or 2 sprigs basil, oregano, or your favorite herb

2 cups extra-virgin olive oil, divided

½ teaspoon black peppercorns

1. Combine the garlic, olives, herbs, and ½ cup of the oil in a small saucepan.
2. Heat gently over medium heat for 5 to 7 minutes, or until the garlic turns golden.
3. Remove the pan from the heat and let cool. Strain the oil through a fine cheesecloth and discard the garlic, olives, and herbs. Add the strained oil to the remaining 1½ cups oil. Add the peppercorns and place in a sterilized jar or bottle. Refrigerate for up to 2 weeks.

Nut-Flavored Oil (*makes 2 cups*)

1 cup walnuts, hazelnuts, or almonds

2 cups extra-virgin olive oil, divided

1. In a blender or food processor, combine the nuts and ½ cup of the oil. Blend or process until the nuts are finely chopped. Add to the remaining 1½ cups oil and place in a sterilized jar or bottle.
2. Cover and refrigerate for 10 days. Strain the nuts from the oil and return the oil to the refrigerator. Use within 1 month.

NUT TOPPINGS

Use these mixed-nut toppings to complement your favorite salads, fruit crisps, or coffee cakes—or snack on them straight from the dish!

Basic Sweet Nuts *(makes ¾ cup)*

¼ cup chopped walnuts
¼ cup chopped pecans
¼ cup chopped Brazil nuts
½ teaspoon cinnamon
1 tablespoon agave nectar

1. Preheat the oven to 350°F. Line a small baking sheet with foil and coat the foil with cooking spray.
2. Combine the walnuts, pecans, Brazil nuts, and cinnamon in a medium bowl. Add the agave nectar and toss to coat.
3. Spread the nut mixture evenly on the prepared sheet and bake for 8 to 10 minutes.
4. Cool completely and store in a resealable plastic bag.

Chocolate Dessert Nuts *(makes 1 cup)*

1½ tablespoons brown sugar
1 tablespoon Dutch process cocoa or 2 tablespoons semisweet chocolate chips, finely chopped
¼ teaspoon cinnamon
½ cup chopped pecans
½ cup chopped hazelnuts
2 teaspoons canola oil

1. Preheat the oven to 350°F. Line a small baking sheet with foil and coat the foil with cooking spray.
2. Combine the sugar, cocoa or chocolate chips, and cinnamon in a small bowl. Add the pecans, hazelnuts, and oil and toss to coat.
3. Spread the nut mixture evenly on the prepared sheet and bake for 8 to 10 minutes.
4. Cool completely and store in a resealable plastic bag.

BBQ Snack Nuts *(makes 1 cup)*

1 teaspoon chili powder
½ teaspoon ground cumin
¼ teaspoon dry mustard
⅛ teaspoon cayenne pepper
½ cup almonds
½ cup peanuts
2 teaspoons canola oil

1. Preheat the over to 350°F. Line a small baking sheet with foil and coat the foil with cooking spray.
2. Combine the spices in a medium bowl. Add the nuts and oil and toss to coat.
3. Spread the nut mixture evenly on the prepared sheet and bake for 8 to 10 minutes.
4. Cool completely and store in a resealable plastic bag.

HOMEMADE SEASONING MIXES

The spice aisle is teeming with dozens of seasoning mixes that are quick, convenient—and frequently contain gluten. If you keep a good supply of basic herbs and spices on hand, though, you can whip up your own mixes for a fraction of the cost. Store each blend tightly covered in a cool, dry place.

Curry Powder (*makes ½ cup*)

- ¼ cup ground coriander
- 1½ tablespoons ground turmeric
- 1 tablespoon ground fenugreek
- 1 tablespoon ground cumin
- 1 teaspoon ground cardamom
- 1 teaspoon ground ginger
- 1 teaspoon ground cinnamon
- 1 teaspoon allspice
- ⅛ teaspoon ground red pepper (or more to taste)

Cajun Spice Mix (*makes ⅔ cup*)

- 2 tablespoons paprika
- 2 tablespoons freshly ground black pepper
- 1 tablespoon garlic powder
- 2 teaspoons red-pepper flakes
- 2 teaspoons dried thyme
- 2 teaspoons dried oregano
- 2 teaspoons onion powder
- 2 teaspoons mustard powder

Middle Eastern Spice Mix (*makes ⅔ cup*)

- 2 tablespoons freshly ground black pepper
- 1½ tablespoons ground cumin
- 1 tablespoon ground coriander
- 1 tablespoon salt
- 1½ teaspoons ground cardamom
- ¾ teaspoon ground cloves

Italian Spice Mix (*makes ⅓ cup*)

- 2 tablespoons dried basil
- 2 teaspoons dried marjoram
- 2 teaspoons thyme
- 2 teaspoons rosemary
- 2 teaspoons oregano
- 1 teaspoon garlic powder

Mexican Spice Mix (*makes ¼ cup*)

- 2 tablespoons chili powder
- 1 tablespoon paprika
- 1 teaspoon ground cumin
- ½ teaspoon dried oregano
- ½ teaspoon garlic powder
- ¼ teaspoon onion powder
- ¼ teaspoon ground chipotle chile pepper
- ¼ teaspoon salt

Jamaican Jerk Spice Mix

- 2 teaspoons cayenne pepper
- 2 tablespoons ground allspice
- 2 tablespoons dried onions
- 4 teaspoons salt
- 1½ teaspoons onion powder
- 1½ teaspoons dried thyme
- 1½ teaspoons dried mustard seed, crushed
- 1 teaspoon dried pepper
- 1 teaspoon dried nutmeg
- ⅛ teaspoon ground cloves

Baking Great Gluten-Free Goodies

Gluten-free baking is both art and science, and goodies like the cakes, cookies, quick breads, and muffins in Chapters 12 and 13 are scrumptious when you use a few gluten-free baking tricks of the trade. Armed with the tips below, you'll be turning out yummy gluten-free treats in no time. (If your kitchen isn't 100 percent gluten free, follow the tips in "Avoid Cross-Contamination in the Kitchen" on page 63, too.)

Use more than one flour. Most gluten-free grains are ground into flour; so are potatoes, tapioca, nuts, and beans. Each of these gluten-free flours has unique properties that affect the finished item's texture and flavor. Gluten-free experts agree: Using a combination of gluten-free flours results in a tastier finished product. Experiment and taste as you bake—you'll soon gain a knack for using the right flour combinations. For example, a combination of bean and sorghum flours can produce a moist, delicious chocolate cake.

Whip it good. Bakers know never to overbeat wheat dough—the gluten bonds become too strong and elastic, resulting in a tough loaf. But you want to beat gluten-free dough. It lightens the dough by introducing air bubbles. Be sure to beat for the full time called for in recipes. To make the process easier, use a heavy-duty stand mixer, rather than the handheld variety.

Oil up. Gluten-free doughs and batters tend to be on the sticky side, so oil your hands before you work them. You can wet them with water, too.

Stamp out steam. Because gluten-free doughs are often moist, breads or pizza dough can turn out mushy if they emit too much steam as they bake. To crisp them up, bake pizza dough on a pizza stone. When you bake bread, remove it from the loaf pan when it's firm enough to hold its shape (about two-thirds of the way through baking), and finish baking it on your oven rack or a preheated pizza stone.

Give flours the deep freeze. Many gluten-free flours, including those made with legumes, nuts, and whole grains, spoil faster than regular flour because they contain more good fats. To keep these fattier flours fresh, keep them in the freezer in resealable plastic bags (squeeze out excess air) or a plastic container with a tight-fitting lid.

BREAKFAST

Blueberry-Almond Breakfast Pudding

■ PREP TIME: 10 MINUTES ■ TOTAL TIME: 25 MINUTES ■ MAKES 4 SERVINGS ■ MUFA: ALMONDS

You can substitute almond milk or 2% milk for the soy milk. If you like, walnuts or pecans can be used in place of the almonds.

½ cup sliced almonds, divided	1 tablespoon chia seeds
4 cups water	1 teaspoon ground cinnamon
Pinch of salt	1 cup vanilla soy milk
2 cups gluten-free rolled oats	1 cup blueberries
2 tablespoons maple syrup	

1. In a small dry skillet, toast the almonds over medium heat for 2 to 3 minutes, shaking the pan often, or until lightly toasted. Transfer the almonds to a cutting board to cool, then coarsely chop.

2. In a medium saucepan over high heat, bring the water and salt to a boil. Gradually stir in the oats, maple syrup, chia seeds, and cinnamon and bring to a boil. Reduce the heat and cook, stirring occasionally, for 10 minutes, or until the oatmeal is tender. Stir in the soy milk, blueberries, and ¼ cup of the almonds.

3. Divide the oatmeal among 4 bowls and sprinkle each serving with 1 tablespoon of the remaining almonds.

Nutrition per serving: 330 calories, 12 g protein, 50 g carbohydrates, 10 g total fat, 1 g saturated fat, 8 g fiber, 106 mg sodium

Make It a FLAT BELLY DIET MEAL
Serve with 1 cup fat-free milk (80).
TOTAL MEAL: 410 calories

Orange and Dried Cherry Porridge

Millet is a small, round grain that is easily digested and easy on your blood sugar. It is loaded with fiber and B-complex vitamins. Toasting the millet for a few minutes brings out its nutty, mild flavor.

⅔ cup millet	2 tablespoons packed brown sugar
2 cups water	¼ teaspoon ground allspice
½ cup orange juice	1 cup 2% milk
½ cup dried cherries	½ cup chopped pistachios

1. In a medium saucepan, toast the millet over medium heat for 3 minutes, stirring often, or until the millet is fragrant and just begins to pop.

2. Gradually stir in the water, orange juice, dried cherries, brown sugar, and allspice and bring to a boil. Reduce the heat to low, cover, and cook, stirring occasionally, for 25 to 30 minutes, or until the millet is tender and the liquid is absorbed.

3. Stir in the milk and heat through. Top each serving with 2 tablespoons of the pistachios.

Nutrition per serving: 332 calories, 10 g protein, 54 g carbohydrates, 9 g total fat, 1.5 g saturated fat, 9 g fiber, 98 mg sodium

Make It a
FLAT
BELLY
DIET
MEAL
}

Serve with 1 cup fat-free milk (80).
TOTAL MEAL: 412 calories

Chocolate–Peanut Butter Stuffed French Toast with Strawberry Sauce

▓ PREP TIME: 15 MINUTES ▓ TOTAL TIME: 30 MINUTES ▓ MAKES 4 SERVINGS
▓ MUFA: CHOCOLATE, PEANUT BUTTER

The strawberry sauce that accompanies this decadent French toast can be turned into a triple berry sauce, if you like. Simply reduce the amount of strawberries to 1 cup and add ½ cup blueberries and ½ cup raspberries instead.

2 cups sliced strawberries	8 slices gluten-free sandwich bread
1 tablespoon sugar	1 egg
1 teaspoon grated orange peel	3 egg whites
½ cup semisweet chocolate chips	1 teaspoon pure vanilla extract
¼ cup peanut butter	1 tablespoon butter

1. In a medium bowl, combine the strawberries, sugar, and orange peel. Set aside.

2. In a saucepan or microwaveable bowl, melt the chocolate chips. Stir in the peanut butter until well mixed. Spread 2 tablespoons of the mixture on each of 4 bread slices and cover with the remaining 4 slices, making sandwiches.

3. In a large bowl, whisk together the egg, egg whites, and vanilla until blended. Working one at a time, dip both sides of each sandwich in the egg mixture and set on a plate.

4. In a large nonstick skillet, melt the butter over medium heat. Wait for the foam to subside, then add the sandwiches and cook for 4 minutes per side, or until golden and cooked through. Serve hot, topped with the reserved strawberry mixture.

Nutrition per serving: 432 calories, 14 g protein, 49 g carbohydrates, 23 g total fat, 7.5 g saturated fat, 5 g fiber, 439 mg sodium

Make It a FLAT BELLY DIET MEAL   A single serving of this recipe counts as a Flat Belly Diet meal without any add-ons!

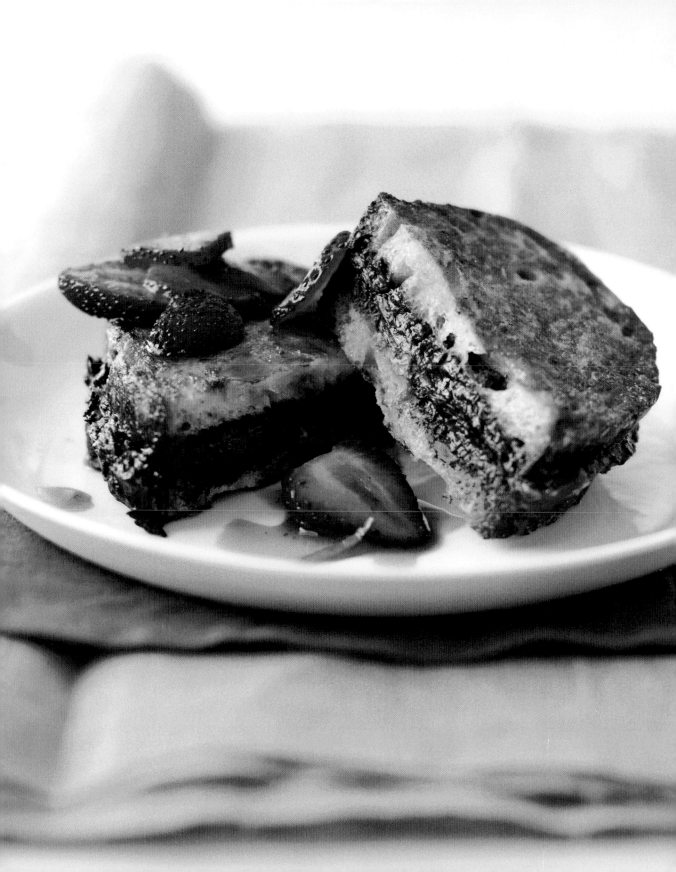

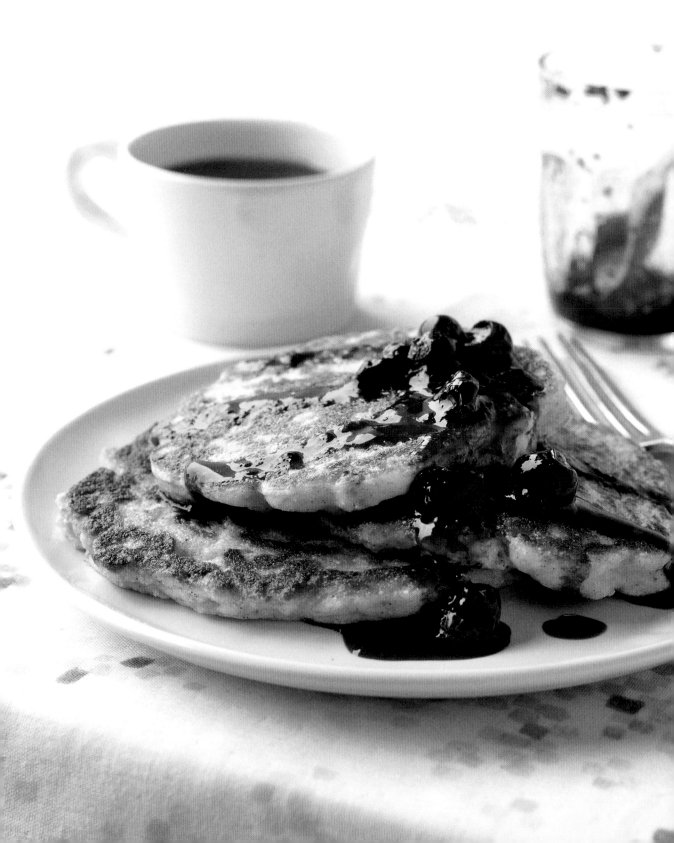

Cornmeal Flapjacks with Blueberry Syrup

■ PREP TIME: 10 MINUTES ■ TOTAL TIME: 30 MINUTES ■ MAKES 4 SERVINGS ■ MUFA: WALNUTS

For best results, stir the batter just until blended. Overmixing will toughen the combined flours. Buttermilk adds tang and makes these flapjacks light and fluffy.

SYRUP

2 cups blueberries
$\frac{1}{4}$ cup water
1 tablespoon sugar

PANCAKES

$\frac{1}{2}$ cup sorghum flour
$\frac{1}{4}$ cup white rice flour
$\frac{1}{4}$ cup tapioca flour

$\frac{1}{4}$ cup cornmeal
$1\frac{1}{2}$ teaspoons baking powder
1 teaspoon xanthan gum
$\frac{1}{4}$ teaspoon salt
$1\frac{1}{4}$ cups buttermilk
1 egg
1 egg white
1 tablespoon canola oil
$\frac{1}{2}$ cup finely chopped walnuts

1. **To make the syrup:** In a medium saucepan over medium-high heat, bring the blueberries, water, and sugar to a boil. Reduce the heat to medium and cook, stirring occasionally, for 10 minutes, or until the mixture bubbles and thickens slightly. Set aside.

2. **To make the pancakes:** In a medium bowl, combine the sorghum flour, white rice flour, tapioca flour, cornmeal, baking powder, xanthan gum, and salt. In a small bowl, whisk together the buttermilk, egg, egg white, and oil. Stir the buttermilk mixture and the walnuts into the flour mixture just until combined.

3. Coat a large nonstick skillet or griddle with cooking spray and heat over medium heat. Drop the batter by scant $\frac{1}{4}$ cupfuls onto the skillet and cook for 3 minutes, or until bubbles begin to appear and the edges look cooked. Turn the pancakes and cook for 2 to 3 minutes. Transfer to a plate and keep warm. Repeat with the remaining batter, making a total of 12 pancakes.

4. Divide the pancakes among 4 plates and serve with the reserved blueberry syrup.

Nutrition per serving: 385 calories, 11 g protein, 54 g carbohydrates, 16 g total fat, 2 g saturated fat, 6 g fiber, 445 mg sodium

Make It a
FLAT
BELLY
DIET
MEAL
} A single serving of this recipe counts as a Flat Belly Diet meal without any add-ons!

Almond Waffles with Tropical Fruit Salsa

■ PREP TIME: 10 MINUTES ■ TOTAL TIME: 30 MINUTES ■ MAKES 4 SERVINGS ■ MUFA: ALMONDS

The batter can be made ahead of time and stored, covered, overnight in the refrigerator. While the waffle iron is heating, let the batter stand at room temperature. Add a little more milk if the batter is too thick.

SALSA
1 mango, chopped
2 kiwifruit, chopped
2 teaspoons honey
1 teaspoon lime juice

WAFFLES
3/4 cup brown rice flour
1/2 cup almond meal

1/4 cup sorghum flour
1 teaspoon baking powder
1 teaspoon xanthan gum
1 egg
1 egg white
1/2 cup fat-free milk
2 teaspoons sugar
1 tablespoon canola oil
1/2 cup sliced almonds, toasted

1. **To make the salsa:** In a large bowl, combine the mango, kiwifruit, honey, and lime juice until well mixed. Set aside.

2. **To make the waffles:** In a medium bowl, whisk together the brown rice flour, almond meal, sorghum flour, baking powder, and xanthan gum. In a small bowl, whisk together the egg, egg white, milk, sugar, and oil. Stir into the flour mixture until well combined.

3. Preheat a waffle iron and lightly coat with cooking spray. Pour the batter into the waffle iron according to the manufacturer's directions. Close and cook for 3 to 5 minutes, or until the steaming stops and the waffle is crisp. Repeat to make 4 waffles.

4. Divide the waffles among 4 plates. Top each serving with 1/2 cup of the reserved salsa and 2 tablespoons of the almonds.

Nutrition per serving: 418 calories, 13 g protein, 55 g carbohydrates, 19 g total fat, 2 g saturated fat, 8 g fiber, 177 mg sodium

Make It a
FLAT
BELLY
DIET
MEAL
} A single serving of this recipe counts as a Flat Belly Diet meal without any add-ons!

Grab-and-Go Breakfast Cups

■ PREP TIME: 10 MINUTES ■ TOTAL TIME: 35 MINUTES ■ MAKES 4 SERVINGS ■ MUFA: OLIVES

These portable little breakfast cups freeze beautifully. Make a batch ahead of time, cool, then wrap individually in waxed paper, then plastic wrap. Place in a resealable food storage bag and freeze for up to 1 month. To reheat, warm in a 325°F oven for 10 minutes or until heated through.

8 eggs

3 tablespoons reduced-fat crumbled feta cheese

2 tablespoons finely chopped pimientos, drained

2 tablespoons chopped fresh dill

½ cup pitted and chopped kalamata olives, divided

1. Preheat the oven to 375°F. Coat four 6-ounce ramekins or custard cups with cooking spray.

2. In a large bowl, whisk the eggs until frothy. Stir in the cheese, pimientos, dill, and ¼ cup of the olives until well combined.

3. Divide the egg mixture among the ramekins. Place the ramekins on a small rimmed baking sheet. Bake for 20 to 25 minutes, or until the filling is set and slightly puffed. Top each serving with 1 tablespoon of the remaining olives.

Nutrition per serving: 271 calories, 15 g protein, 5 g carbohydrates, 21 g total fat, 5 g saturated fat, 1 g fiber, 883 mg sodium

Make It a
FLAT
BELLY
DIET
MEAL
} Serve with ½ toasted gluten-free English muffin (135) topped with 1 tablespoon apple butter (29).
TOTAL MEAL: 435 calories

Red Flannel Hash and Eggs

■ PREP TIME: 10 MINUTES ■ TOTAL TIME: 30 MINUTES ■ MAKES 4 SERVINGS ■ MUFA: OLIVE OIL

Here is a great way to use leftovers. Any combination of meat and vegetables can be used. Substitute chopped cooked turkey or ham for the corned beef. Or, to make this meatless, use 1 cup cubed firm tofu in place of the corned beef.

¼ cup olive oil

1 large Yukon gold potato, peeled and cut into small cubes

4 scallions, thinly sliced

2 cloves garlic, minced

1 cup chopped cooked beets

6 ounces gluten-free lean corned beef, chopped

2 tablespoons chopped fresh parsley

¼ teaspoon ground black pepper

4 eggs

1. In a large nonstick skillet over medium-high heat, warm the oil. Cook the potato for 8 minutes, stirring occasionally, or until the potato is tender and lightly browned. Add the scallions and garlic and cook for 1 minute, or until the scallions are softened. Add the beets, corned beef, parsley, and pepper. Cook, stirring occasionally, for 5 minutes, or until heated through.

2. Meanwhile, bring a medium skillet of water to a simmer. Break the eggs, one at a time, into a custard cup or ramekin. Carefully slip each egg into the simmering water. Cook for 3 to 4 minutes, or until desired degree of doneness. Carefully remove the poached eggs with a slotted spoon.

3. To serve, divide the hash among 4 plates. Top each serving with a poached egg.

Nutrition per serving: 383 calories, 16 g protein, 20 g carbohydrates, 27 g total fat, 6 g saturated fat, 3 g fiber, 636 mg sodium

Make It a
FLAT
BELLY
DIET
MEAL

A single serving of this recipe counts as a Flat Belly Diet meal without any add-ons!

Pan-Fried Cheesy Polenta

■ PREP TIME: 10 MINUTES ■ TOTAL TIME: 1 HOUR 15 MINUTES ■ MAKES 4 SERVINGS
■ MUFA: CANOLA OIL

To make clean cuts when cutting the polenta into rectangles, use a sharp knife lightly coated with cooking spray.

$\frac{1}{4}$ cup canola oil, divided	3 cups water
1 onion, finely chopped	$\frac{1}{4}$ teaspoon salt
2 cloves garlic, minced	$\frac{3}{4}$ cup gluten-free instant polenta
1 teaspoon chopped fresh rosemary	1 cup shredded reduced-fat sharp Cheddar cheese

1. Coat an 8" x 8" baking pan with cooking spray.

2. In a small nonstick skillet over medium-high heat, warm 3 tablespoons of the oil. Cook the onion and garlic, stirring occasionally, for 5 minutes, or until softened. Remove from the heat and stir in the rosemary. Set aside.

3. In a medium saucepan over medium-high heat, bring the water and salt to a boil. Whisk in the polenta in a slow, steady stream. Reduce the heat to medium and cook, stirring constantly with a wooden spoon, for 3 to 5 minutes, or until the polenta thickens. Remove from the heat and stir in the cheese and the reserved onion mixture. Pour into the prepared pan, smooth with a spatula, and let stand at room temperature for 35 to 40 minutes, or until completely cooled and set.

4. Turn the cooled polenta out onto a cutting board and cut into 8 rectangles. Wipe out the skillet and heat 2 teaspoons of the remaining oil over medium-high heat. Cook 4 polenta rectangles for 3 minutes per side, or until lightly browned. Transfer to a plate to keep warm and repeat with the remaining 1 teaspoon oil and polenta.

Nutrition per serving: 367 calories, 10 g protein, 40 g carbohydrates, 20 g total fat, 5 g saturated fat, 2 g fiber, 382 mg sodium

Make It a
FLAT
BELLY
DIET
MEAL

Serve with 1 cup sliced strawberries (47).
TOTAL MEAL: 414 calories

Black Olive Tapenade

■ PREP TIME: 5 MINUTES ■ TOTAL TIME: 5 MINUTES ■ MAKES 12 SERVINGS ■ MUFA: OLIVES

This rich olive paste is a versatile ingredient for many Flat Belly Diet recipes and is incredibly easy to make at home.

2 cups Niçoise olives, pitted

2 teaspoons capers, rinsed and drained

3 cloves garlic

2 tablespoons olive oil

1 tablespoon freshly squeezed lemon juice

¼ teaspoon ground black pepper

1. In a food processor, combine the olives, capers, and garlic. Pulse until coarsely chopped. Combine the oil and lemon juice in a measuring cup. With the machine running, add the oil mixture through the feed tube to blend into a rough paste. Add the pepper and pulse to combine.

2. Transfer to an airtight container. Refrigerate for up to 2 weeks.

Nutrition per serving: 60 calories, 0 g protein, 2 g carbohydrates, 5 g total fat, 0.5 g saturated fat, 1 g fiber, 270 mg sodium

Make It a
FLAT
BELLY
DIET
MEAL

Serve spread on 2 slices gluten-free bread (100) topped with 2 eggs scrambled in a nonstick pan coated with cooking spray (156), and 1 slice reduced-fat provolone (77).

TOTAL MEAL: 393 calories

Frittata with Smoked Salmon and Dill

■ PREP TIME: 10 MINUTES ■ TOTAL TIME: 25 MINUTES ■ MAKES 6 SERVINGS
■ MUFA: BLACK OLIVE TAPENADE

Other MUFA fillings, such as pesto, or topping each serving with ¼ cup chopped avocado in place of the tapenade, would work well here, too.

2 teaspoons olive oil

2 shallots, thinly sliced

6 egg whites

4 eggs

¼ cup cold water

1 tablespoon chopped fresh dill

½ teaspoon salt

Ground black pepper

2 ounces thinly sliced smoked salmon, cut into ½"-wide pieces

¾ cup Black Olive Tapenade (opposite page) or store-bought gluten-free tapenade

1. Preheat the oven to 350°F. In a heavy ovenproof skillet over medium-high heat, warm the oil. Cook the shallots, stirring, for 2 minutes, or until soft.

2. In a medium bowl, whisk together the egg whites, eggs, water, dill, and salt. Season with pepper. Pour the mixture into the skillet and lay the salmon pieces on top. Cook, stirring, for 2 minutes, or until partially set.

3. Transfer to the oven and cook for 6 to 8 minutes, or until firm, golden, and puffed. Slide the frittata onto a plate. Spread 2 tablespoons of the tapenade on each of 6 plates and place a slice of frittata on top.

Nutrition per serving: 154 calories, 11 g protein, 7 g carbohydrates, 10 g total fat, 2 g saturated fat, 1 g fiber, 584 mg sodium

Make It a
FLAT
BELLY
DIET
MEAL

Serve with 2 ounces gluten-free lean Italian turkey sausage (70) and a Pomegranate-Peach Smoothie (page 94), but omit the flaxseed oil (177). TOTAL MEAL: 401 calories

Huevos Rancheros

■ PREP TIME: 15 MINUTES ■ TOTAL TIME: 40 MINUTES ■ MAKES 4 SERVINGS ■ MUFA: AVOCADO

A recent study found that eating eggs for breakfast at least 5 days a week can help you lose more weight—especially around your middle. Study participants also reported having more energy.

2 teaspoons olive oil	1 can (15 ounces) no-salt-added pinto beans, rinsed and drained
1 red bell pepper, cut into thin strips	½ cup gluten-free low-sodium chicken broth
4 scallions, sliced	
1 jalapeño chile pepper, seeded and finely chopped (wear plastic gloves when handling)	4 eggs
	1 avocado, sliced
2 cloves garlic, minced	4 tablespoons 0% plain Greek yogurt
1 teaspoon ground cumin	4 tablespoons gluten-free medium or mild tomatillo salsa

1. In a large nonstick skillet over medium-high heat, warm the oil. Cook the bell pepper, scallions, chile pepper, garlic, and cumin for 8 minutes, stirring occasionally, or until softened. Add the beans and broth and bring to a boil. Reduce the heat to medium, and cook, stirring occasionally, for 8 minutes, or until most of the broth is evaporated. With the back of a wooden spoon, smash the beans until they are lumpy.

2. Use the back of the spoon to make 4 indentations in the bean mixture. Working one at a time, break each egg into a custard cup and pour into each indentation. Cover and cook for 8 minutes, or until the eggs are cooked to the desired doneness.

3. Scoop each portion of the egg-topped bean mixture onto a plate. Scatter the avocado slices over and around the beans. Top each serving with 1 tablespoon of the yogurt and 1 tablespoon of the salsa.

Nutrition per serving: 335 calories, 16 g protein, 39 g carbohydrates, 14 g total fat, 3 g saturated fat, 10 g fiber, 122 mg sodium

Make It a FLAT BELLY DIET MEAL

Serve with a toasted 7" gluten-free corn tortilla (70).
TOTAL MEAL: 405 calories

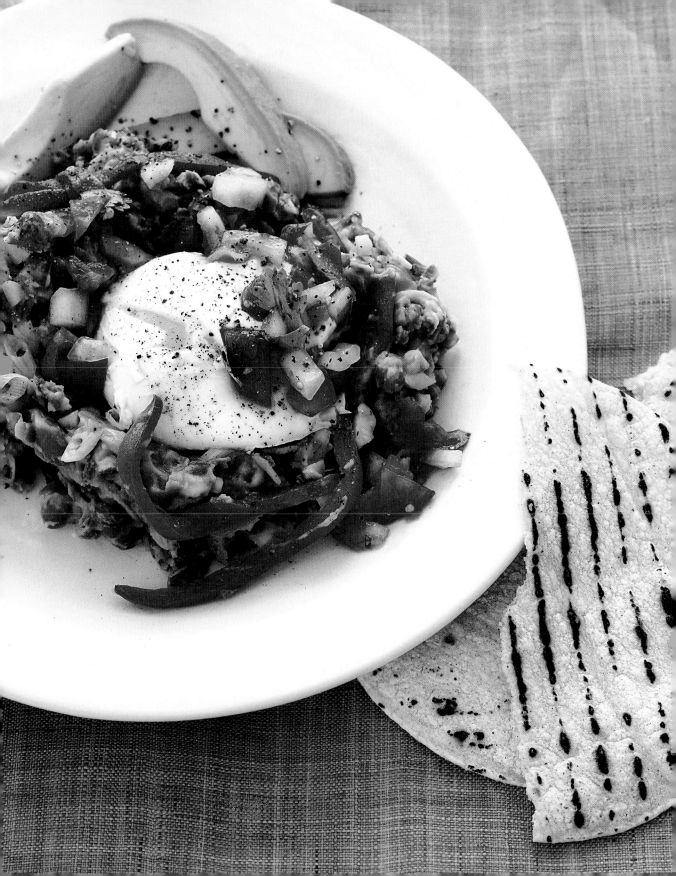

Pesto

■ PREP TIME: 10 MINUTES ■ TOTAL TIME: 10 MINUTES ■ MAKES 24 SERVINGS

This sauce provides the perfect reason to grow fresh basil. Make several batches when this fragrant herb is in season and freeze what you don't need.

½ cup pine nuts	1 teaspoon salt
6 cups packed fresh basil	¼ teaspoon ground black pepper
1 clove garlic	½ cup extra-virgin olive oil
½ cup grated Parmesan cheese	

1. In a large nonstick skillet, toast the pine nuts over medium heat, stirring often, for 3 to 4 minutes, or until lightly browned and fragrant. Tip onto a plate and let cool.

2. In a food processor, combine the pine nuts, basil, garlic, cheese, salt, and pepper. Pulse until coarsely chopped. With the machine running, add the oil through the feed tube to blend into a rough paste.

3. Transfer to an airtight container. Refrigerate for up to 1 week.

Nutrition per serving: 71 calories, 1 g protein, 1 g carbohydrates, 7 g total fat, 1 g saturated fat, 1 g fiber, 123 mg sodium

Make It a FLAT BELLY DIET MEAL

Serve with ½ cup cooked gluten-free elbow pasta (101) tossed with 4 ounces grilled chicken breast (187), 2 sun-dried tomatoes packed in oil (30), and 1½ cups fresh spinach (6).
TOTAL MEAL: 395 calories

Broccoli and Pesto Omelet

▓ PREP TIME: 10 MINUTES ▓ TOTAL TIME: 25 MINUTES ▓ MAKES 4 SERVINGS ▓ MUFA: PESTO

Broccoli is high in folate, an essential B vitamin for those with celiac disease or non-celiac gluten sensitivity.

2 cups broccoli florets
1 tablespoon olive oil
2 cloves garlic, minced
¼ teaspoon red-pepper flakes
½ teaspoon salt, divided
3 eggs

3 egg whites
½ cup 1% milk
½ cup shredded part-skim mozzarella cheese
4 tablespoons Pesto (opposite page) or store-bought gluten-free pesto

1. Place a steamer basket in a large saucepan with 2″ of water. Bring to a boil over high heat, add the broccoli, and steam for 4 minutes, or until tender-crisp. Drain under cold running water and drain again. Pat broccoli dry with paper towels.

2. In a large nonstick skillet over medium-high heat, warm the oil. Add the broccoli, garlic, red-pepper flakes, and ¼ teaspoon of the salt. Cook for 3 minutes, or until fragrant.

3. Meanwhile, in a large bowl, whisk together the eggs, egg whites, milk, and the remaining ¼ teaspoon salt until well blended.

4. Pour the egg mixture into the skillet and cook, gently lifting the edges to let the uncooked portion flow underneath, for 7 minutes, or until the eggs are partially set.

5. Sprinkle the cheese evenly over half of the omelet. Fold over the other half of the omelet to cover the cheese. Cut into 4 wedges. Top each serving with 1 tablespoon of the pesto.

Nutrition per serving: 241 calories, 16 g protein, 6 g carbohydrates, 18 g total fat, 5.5 g saturated fat, 2 g fiber, 601 mg sodium

Make It a FLAT BELLY DIET MEAL

Serve with 1 cup roasted baby red potatoes (151).
TOTAL MEAL: 392 calories

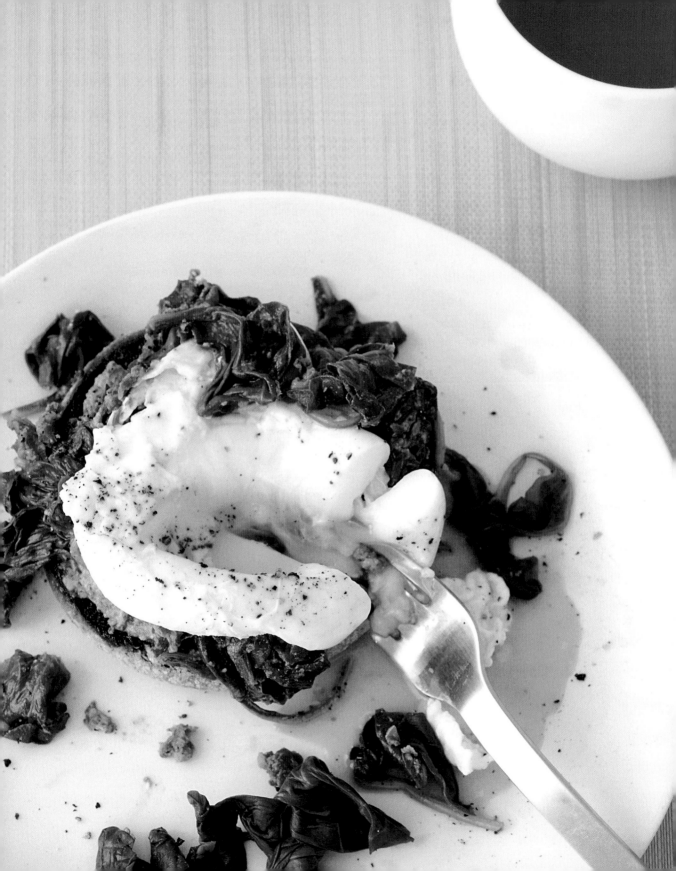

Poached Eggs with Spinach and Sun-Dried Tomato Pesto

■ PREP TIME: 10 MINUTES ■ TOTAL TIME: 20 MINUTES ■ MAKES 4 SERVINGS ■ MUFA: PESTO

Fresh eggs, used within a week of purchase, are best for poaching because the whites are still firm and cling to the yolk better. This gives the poached egg a neat, uniform shape. The whites of older eggs are thinner and tend to feather out into the poaching liquid.

⅓ cup 0% plain Greek yogurt	Pinch of salt
¼ cup gluten-free sun-dried tomato pesto	4 eggs
1 teaspoon olive oil	2 gluten-free English muffins, split and toasted
1 package (9 ounces) baby spinach	Ground black pepper
1 teaspoon vinegar	

1. In a small bowl, combine the yogurt and pesto until blended.

2. In a large nonstick skillet over medium-high heat, warm the oil. Cook the spinach, stirring often, for 2 to 3 minutes, or until wilted. Remove from the heat. Stir in ¼ cup of the yogurt mixture until blended. Cover and keep warm. Set the remaining yogurt mixture aside.

3. Meanwhile, bring a medium skillet with 1" of water to a boil over high heat. Add the vinegar and salt and reduce the heat to a simmer. Break the eggs, one at a time, into a custard cup or ramekin. Carefully slip each egg into the simmering water. Cook for 3 to 4 minutes, or until desired degree of doneness. Carefully remove the poached eggs with a slotted spoon. Stir 1 tablespoon of the poaching liquid into the reserved yogurt mixture to thin.

4. Place a muffin half on each of 4 plates. Top each muffin half evenly with the spinach mixture and a poached egg. Spoon the yogurt mixture evenly over each egg and grind some pepper over the top.

Nutrition per serving: 213 calories, 11 g protein, 27 g carbohydrates, 7 g total fat, 2 g saturated fat, 4 g fiber, 456 mg sodium

Make It a FLAT BELLY DIET MEAL
Serve with 1 cup fresh pineapple slices (97) and ¾ cup fresh orange juice (84).
TOTAL MEAL: 394 calories

Potato and Pepper Torta

■ PREP TIME: 15 MINUTES ■ TOTAL TIME: 45 MINUTES ■ MAKES 4 SERVINGS ■ MUFA: OLIVE OIL

Green frying peppers, also known as Cubanelles, are long, thin, and banana shaped. They have a mild sweet flavor and are easy to digest.

¼ cup olive oil	3 eggs
3 green frying peppers, seeded and chopped (about ¾ pound)	3 egg whites
1 sweet onion, thinly sliced	¼ cup water
1 large potato, cooked and cubed	½ teaspoon salt
1 package (5 ounces) baby spinach	½ cup shredded reduced-fat Swiss cheese

1. In a large ovenproof nonstick skillet over medium-high heat, warm the oil. Cook the peppers and onion for 8 minutes, stirring occasionally, or until the peppers are softened. Add the potato and cook for 1 minute. Stir in the spinach, in batches, and cook for 3 minutes, or until wilted.

2. Preheat the oven to 375°F.

3. Meanwhile, in a large bowl, beat the eggs, egg whites, water, and salt until well blended.

4. Pour the egg mixture over the vegetables, stirring to combine. Cook over medium heat for 4 minutes, or until the mixture just begins to set.

5. Sprinkle with the cheese and bake for 15 minutes, or until set. Cut into 4 wedges.

Nutrition per serving: 354 calories, 16 g protein, 35 g carbohydrates, 19 g total fat, 3.5 g saturated fat, 5 g fiber, 662 mg sodium

Make It a FLAT BELLY DIET MEAL

Serve with ½ cup red or green grapes (52).
TOTAL MEAL: 406 calories

Breakfast Tacos with Tomato Guacamole

■ PREP TIME: 10 MINUTES ■ TOTAL TIME: 15 MINUTES ■ MAKES 4 SERVINGS ■ MUFA: AVOCADO

Add 1 tablespoon fresh lime juice to the avocado mixture if you like.

1 Hass avocado, peeled, seeded, and chopped

1 tomato, chopped

¼ small white onion, chopped

1 tablespoon chopped fresh cilantro

2 teaspoons chili powder

½ teaspoon salt, divided

4 eggs

4 egg whites

2 ounces shredded reduced-fat sharp Cheddar cheese

¼ teaspoon ground black pepper

1 teaspoon olive oil

8 gluten-free corn tortillas

1. In a small bowl, combine the avocado, tomato, onion, cilantro, chili powder, and ¼ teaspoon of the salt until well mixed.

2. In a large bowl, whisk together the eggs, egg whites, cheese, pepper, and the remaining ¼ teaspoon salt. In a medium nonstick saucepan over medium-high heat, warm the oil. Add the egg mixture and cook, stirring occasionally, for 3 to 4 minutes, or until scrambled but still moist and creamy.

3. Place the tortillas between paper towels and microwave on high for 15 to 20 seconds, or until warm. Put a tortilla on each of 4 plates and evenly divide the egg mixture among the tortillas. Top each evenly with a second tortilla and the avocado mixture.

Nutrition per serving: 337 calories, 19 g protein, 34 g carbohydrates, 16 g total fat, 4 g saturated fat, 7 g fiber, 516 mg sodium

Make It a FLAT BELLY DIET MEAL

Serve with ¾ cup fresh orange juice (84).
TOTAL MEAL: 421 calories

Apple and Almond Butter Sandwiches

■ PREP TIME: 5 MINUTES ■ TOTAL TIME: 5 MINUTES ■ MAKES 2 SERVINGS
■ MUFA: ALMOND BUTTER

Here is a good way to experiment with different nut butters. Creamy cashew, pistachio, or pecan butter would be equally delicious.

1 gluten-free English muffin, split and toasted

4 tablespoons almond butter

4 teaspoons orange marmalade fruit spread

4 thin apple slices

Place the muffin halves on a work surface. Top each half with 2 tablespoons of the almond butter and 2 teaspoons of the fruit spread. Top each with half of the apple slices and serve open-faced.

Nutrition per serving: 333 calories, 7 g protein, 36 g carbohydrates, 20 g total fat, 2 g saturated fat, 2 g fiber, 353 mg sodium

Make It a
FLAT
BELLY
DIET
MEAL

Serve with 1 cup fat-free milk (83).
TOTAL MEAL: 416 calories

Cinnamon-Raisin Breakfast Sandwich

■ PREP TIME: 5 MINUTES ■ TOTAL TIME: 5 MINUTES ■ MAKES 1 SERVING ■ MUFA: PUMPKIN SEEDS

Gluten-free breads and baked goods have a better shelf life when frozen. Look for them in the freezer section of your supermarket, where there is a wide variety to choose from.

¼ cup 0% plain Greek yogurt	2 slices gluten-free cinnamon-raisin bread, toasted
2 tablespoons pumpkin seeds	½ banana, thinly sliced
1 teaspoon maple syrup	

In a small bowl, combine the yogurt, pumpkin seeds, and syrup until blended. On 1 slice of toast, arrange the banana slices. Top with the yogurt mixture and the remaining slice of toast. Cut in half before serving.

Nutrition per serving: 370 calories, 13 g protein, 60 g carbohydrates, 11 g total fat, 1.5 g saturated fat, 5 g fiber, 264 mg sodium

Make It a
FLAT
BELLY
DIET
MEAL
} A single serving of this recipe counts as a Flat Belly Diet meal without any add-ons!

Crunchy Peanut Butter–Banana Wrap

▓ PREP TIME: 5 MINUTES ▓ TOTAL TIME: 5 MINUTES ▓ MAKES 1 SERVING ▓ MUFA: PEANUT BUTTER

A drizzle of honey replaces unwanted sugar in this sophisticated version of your childhood PB&J.

1 brown rice tortilla (8" diameter)	¼ banana, sliced
2 tablespoons crunchy natural unsalted peanut butter	½ teaspoon honey

Lay the tortilla on a work surface. Spread with the peanut butter. Cover with the banana slices and drizzle with the honey. Roll into a tube. Slice on the diagonal into 4 pieces.

Nutrition per serving: 367 calories, 9 g protein, 41 g carbohydrates, 19 g total fat, 2 g saturated fat, 5 g fiber, 160 mg sodium

Make It a
FLAT
BELLY
DIET
MEAL
A single serving of this recipe counts as a Flat Belly Diet meal without any add-ons!

Blackberry Yogurt Parfaits

▓ PREP TIME: 15 MINUTES ▓ TOTAL TIME: 15 MINUTES ▓ MAKES 2 SERVINGS ▓ MUFA: ALMONDS

For breakfast on the go, assemble the parfaits in portable containers the night before. Sprinkle with the almonds right before eating.

1 cup 0% plain Greek yogurt

1 tablespoon maple syrup

1 teaspoon grated peeled
   fresh ginger

1 cup fresh blackberries

1 navel orange, peeled, sectioned,
   and cut into 1" pieces

¼ cup sliced almonds, toasted

1. In a medium bowl, combine the yogurt, maple syrup, and ginger until blended.

2. Place one-fourth of the blackberries and the orange in the bottoms of 2 parfait glasses. Dollop each with one-fourth of the yogurt mixture. Top with another one-fourth of the blackberries and the orange, followed by the remaining yogurt mixture. Sprinkle each serving with 2 tablespoons of the almonds.

Nutrition per serving: 218 calories, 14 g protein, 30 g carbohydrates, 6 g total fat, 0.5 g saturated fat, 7 g fiber, 45 mg sodium

Make It a FLAT BELLY DIET MEAL

Serve with a gluten-free English muffin (130) topped with 2 teaspoons trans-free margarine (54).
TOTAL MEAL: 402 calories

Pomegranate-Peach Smoothie

▓ PREP TIME: 10 MINUTES ▓ TOTAL TIME: 10 MINUTES ▓ MAKES 1 SERVING ▓ MUFA: FLAXSEED OIL

Pour your smoothie into a thermos and take it with you for a midmorning or afternoon snack. Shake well to recombine before drinking.

1 large peach, pitted and chopped	1 tablespoon flaxseed oil
⅓ cup pomegranate juice	2 teaspoons honey
2 tablespoons 0% plain Greek yogurt	4 ice cubes

In a blender, combine the peach, pomegranate juice, yogurt, oil, honey, and ice cubes. Process until smooth. Pour into a tall glass and serve.

Nutrition per serving: 298 calories, 4 g protein, 43 g carbohydrates, 14 g total fat, 1 g saturated fat, 2 g fiber, 24 mg sodium

Make It a FLAT BELLY DIET MEAL

Serve with 1 piece reduced-fat mozzarella string cheese (70).
TOTAL MEAL: 368 calories

Chocolate–Peanut Butter Smoothie

▓ PREP TIME: 5 MINUTES ▓ TOTAL TIME: 5 MINUTES ▓ MAKES 1 SERVING ▓ MUFA: PEANUT BUTTER

This delicious smoothie is a great midafternoon pick-me-up. It's also delicious with almond or cashew butter instead of peanut butter.

⅔ cup light vanilla soy milk	2 teaspoons unsweetened cocoa powder
¼ small banana	4 ice cubes
2 tablespoons creamy natural peanut butter	

In a blender, combine the soy milk, banana, peanut butter, cocoa powder, and ice cubes. Process until smooth. Pour into a tall glass and serve.

Nutrition per serving: 329 calories, 13 g protein, 29 g carbohydrates, 19 g total fat, 3 g saturated fat, 4 g fiber, 215 mg sodium

Make It a FLAT BELLY DIET MEAL

Serve with 1 medium banana (105).
TOTAL MEAL: 434 calories

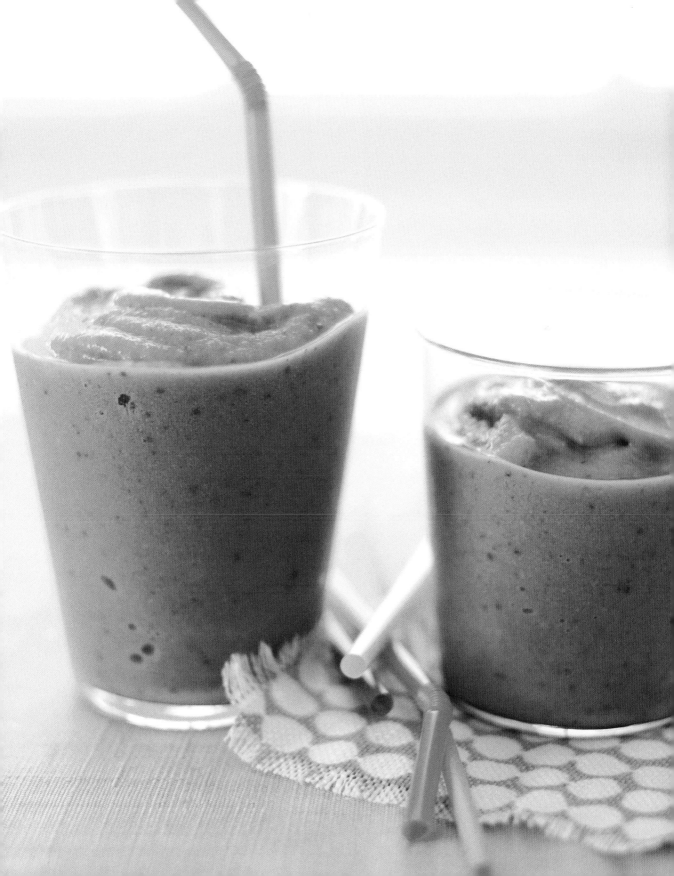

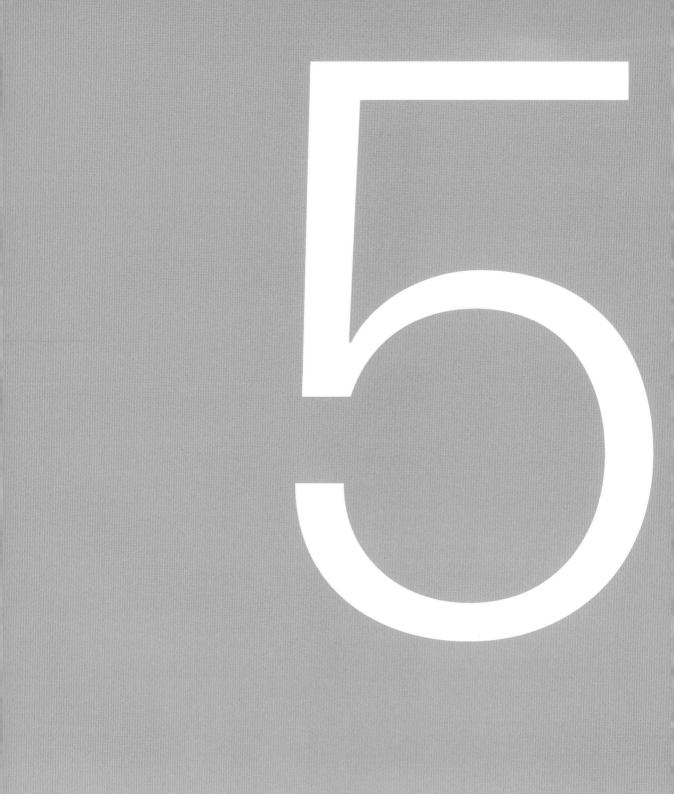

SOUPS AND SANDWICHES

Roast Beef Onion Soup

■ PREP TIME: 15 MINUTES ■ TOTAL TIME: 1 HOUR ■ MAKES 4 SERVINGS (1½ CUPS EACH)
■ MUFA: CANOLA OIL

Every bit as tantalizing as a classic French onion soup, this updated version lowers the sodium considerably using low-sodium roast beef in place of the cheese. Slices of leftover steak work well, too.

¼ cup canola oil
3 large onions, thinly sliced
2 cloves garlic, minced
2 tablespoons balsamic vinegar
4 cups gluten-free low-sodium beef broth

1 teaspoon gluten-free Worcestershire sauce
4 slices (1½ ounces each) thinly sliced low-sodium deli roast beef
1 tablespoon chopped fresh chives (optional)

1. In a large saucepan over medium heat, warm the oil. Cook the onions, stirring occasionally, for 20 to 25 minutes, or until the onions are very tender and begin to caramelize. Stir in the garlic and cook for 1 minute.

2. Add the vinegar and bring to a boil over medium-high heat. Cook, stirring constantly, for 1 minute, or until the vinegar is completely evaporated.

3. Add the broth and Worcestershire sauce and bring to a boil over medium-high heat. Reduce the heat to low, cover, and simmer for 15 minutes, or until the flavors are blended.

4. Ladle the soup into 4 bowls. Garnish each with a slice of roast beef and the chives, if using.

Nutrition per serving: 205 calories, 7 g protein, 13 g carbohydrates, 15 g total fat, 1.5 g saturated fat, 2 g fiber, 169 mg sodium

Make It a
FLAT
BELLY
DIET
MEAL

Serve with ½ cup quinoa (111) mixed with 3 tablespoons raisins (93).
TOTAL MEAL: 409 calories

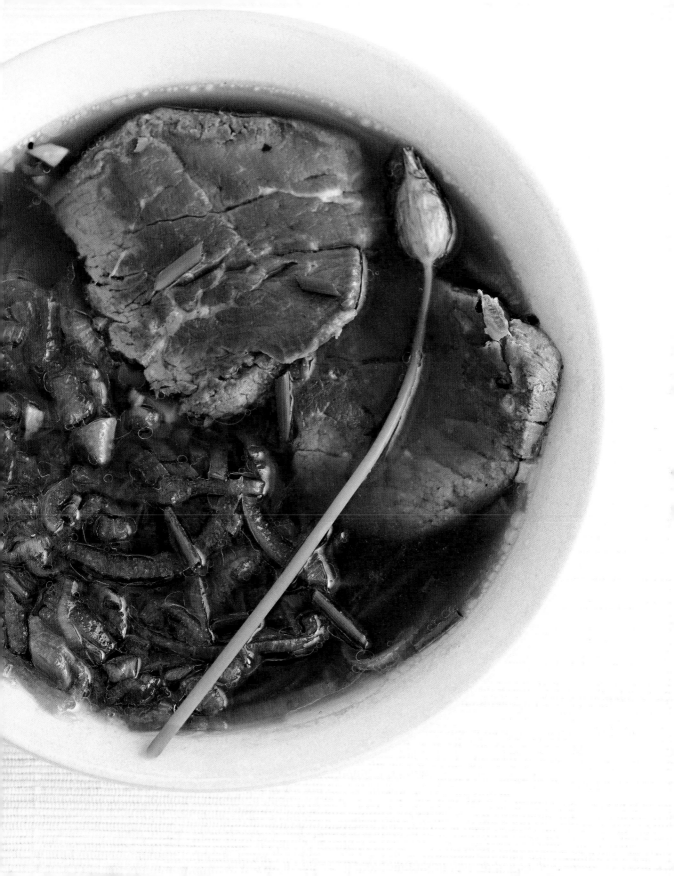

Country Bean and Vegetable Soup

▓ PREP TIME: 15 MINUTES ▓ TOTAL TIME: 2 HOURS 15 MINUTES
▓ MAKES 8 SERVINGS (1½ CUPS EACH) ▓ MUFA: OLIVE OIL

Make this hearty soup a day ahead. It tastes even better the next day.

½ cup olive oil, divided

1 small head green cabbage, chopped

½ large onion, chopped

3 ribs celery, chopped

2 carrots, chopped

2 cloves garlic, minced

3 cans (14.5 ounces each) gluten-free low-sodium vegetable broth, divided

½ cup dried white beans

1½ teaspoons chopped fresh thyme or ½ teaspoon dried

1½ teaspoons chopped fresh sage or ½ teaspoon dried

½ pound green beans, cut into 1" pieces

1 medium zucchini, halved lengthwise and sliced into half moons

1. Warm ¼ cup of the oil in a large saucepan over medium-high heat. Add the cabbage, onion, celery, carrots, and garlic and cook, stirring occasionally, for 10 minutes, or until the vegetables are softened. Add 2 cans of the broth, the beans, thyme, and sage and bring to a boil. Reduce the heat to low, cover, and simmer for 1 to 1½ hours, or until the beans are almost tender, adding the remaining broth if the soup becomes too thick.

2. Stir in the green beans and zucchini. Partially cover and cook for 20 minutes, or until the white beans are tender.

3. Ladle into 8 bowls. Drizzle each serving with ½ tablespoon of the remaining oil.

Nutrition per serving: 236 calories, 5 g protein, 23 g carbohydrates, 14 g total fat, 2 g saturated fat, 8 g fiber, 163 mg sodium

Make It a
FLAT
BELLY
DIET
MEAL

Serve with ½ Ham and Black Olive Panini (page 109) (158).
TOTAL MEAL: 394 calories

Spicy Sweet Potato–Ginger Soup

▓ PREP TIME: 15 MINUTES ▓ TOTAL TIME: 45 MINUTES ▓ MAKES 8 SERVINGS (1¼ CUPS EACH)
▓ MUFA: AVOCADO

An immersion or stick blender is a handy way to puree this soup. It fits directly
into the saucepan for quick blending and eliminates the need for a food
processor or blender.

1 teaspoon olive oil

2 shallots, thinly sliced

3 tablespoons chopped peeled
fresh ginger

2 cloves garlic, thinly sliced

6 cups gluten-free low-sodium
vegetable broth

4 medium sweet potatoes, peeled
and cubed

1 cup light unsweetened
coconut milk

1 tablespoon lime juice

½ teaspoon salt

¼ cup chopped fresh cilantro

2 Hass avocados, peeled,
pitted, and chopped

1. In a large saucepan over medium-high heat, warm the oil. Cook the shallots, ginger,
and garlic, stirring frequently, for 5 minutes, or until softened. Add the broth and
potatoes and bring to a boil. Reduce the heat and simmer, partially covered, for
20 minutes, or until the potatoes are tender.

2. With a handheld blender, puree the soup until smooth. (Alternately, transfer
the soup to a food processor or blender and pulse, in batches, until smooth. Return the
soup to the saucepan.) Stir in the coconut milk, lime juice, and salt and heat through.

3. Remove from the heat and stir in the cilantro. Top each serving with one-fourth of
the avocado.

Nutrition per serving: 159 calories, 9 g protein, 21 g carbohydrates, 8 g total fat, 2 g saturated fat,
5 g fiber, 295 mg sodium

Make It a
FLAT
BELLY
DIET
MEAL
Serve with Turkey Cutlets with Bacon and Avocado (page 192),
omitting the avocado (158), and 1 cup pitted sweet cherries (90).
TOTAL MEAL: 407 calories

Creamy Southern-Style Peanut Soup

■ PREP TIME: 15 MINUTES ■ TOTAL TIME: 55 MINUTES
■ MAKES 4 SERVINGS (1¼ CUPS EACH) ■ MUFA: PEANUT BUTTER

**This rich and creamy soup is surprisingly satisfying. The peanut butter melts
into the broth, creating a bisquelike consistency, without the cream.**

1 teaspoon canola oil

1 onion, chopped

2 ribs celery, chopped

1 carrot, chopped

1 clove garlic, minced

3 cups gluten-free low-sodium
vegetable broth, divided

½ cup unsalted creamy natural
peanut butter

2 tablespoons lemon juice

2 tablespoons unsalted dry-roasted
peanuts, chopped

1. In a large nonstick saucepot over medium-high heat, warm the oil. Add the onion,
celery, carrot, and garlic and cook, stirring occasionally, for 5 minutes, or until softened.

2. Add 2 cups of the broth and bring to a boil. Reduce the heat to low, cover, and
simmer for 30 minutes, or until the vegetables are very tender.

3. Puree the soup, in batches if necessary, in a food processor or a blender, and return
the soup to the pot. Or leave it in the pot if using an immersion blender, and puree until
smooth.

4. Stir in the peanut butter, lemon juice, and the remaining 1 cup broth. Cook, stirring,
for 5 minutes, or until the peanut butter melts and the flavors are blended.

5. Ladle the soup into 4 bowls and sprinkle each with ½ tablespoon of the peanuts.

Nutrition per serving: 272 calories, 9 g protein, 16 g carbohydrates, 20 g total fat, 2.5 g saturated fat,
5 g fiber, 146 mg sodium

Make It a
FLAT
BELLY
DIET
MEAL

Serve with 3 ounces roasted chicken breast (140).
TOTAL MEAL: 412 calories

Creamy Broccoli and Spinach Soup

■ PREP TIME: 10 MINUTES ■ TOTAL TIME: 45 MINUTES
■ MAKES 4 SERVINGS (1½ CUPS EACH) ■ MUFA: OLIVE OIL

This garden-fresh soup owes its velvety texture to the potato flour and oil added at the end of the cooking process—no dairy here! Don't pass up this soup. Broccoli is one of the most powerful cancer-fighting foods you can eat.

¼ cup olive oil, divided
1 onion, chopped
4 cups gluten-free low-sodium vegetable broth
1 pound broccoli florets, chopped
2 cups baby spinach

3 tablespoons gluten-free potato flour
½ teaspoon salt
¼ teaspoon ground black pepper
Pinch of ground nutmeg

1. In a large saucepot over medium-high heat, warm 1 tablespoon of the oil. Cook the onion, stirring occasionally, for 8 minutes, or until golden brown.

2. Add the broth and broccoli and bring to a boil. Reduce the heat to low, cover, and simmer for 15 minutes, or until the broccoli is tender. Turn off the heat and stir in the spinach until it is wilted. Transfer the mixture to a blender, or leave it in the pot if using an immersion blender, and puree until smooth.

3. Meanwhile, warm the remaining 3 tablespoons oil in a small saucepan over medium heat. Add the potato flour and stir until smooth. Cook, stirring occasionally, for 2 to 3 minutes, or until light brown.

4. Heat the soup in the pot over medium-high heat just until it begins to boil. Reduce the heat to a simmer. Add the potato flour mixture and stir until the soup thickens. Add the salt, pepper, and nutmeg.

Nutrition per serving: 210 calories, 5 g protein, 19 g carbohydrates, 14 g total fat, 2 g saturated fat, 6 g fiber, 486 mg sodium

Make It a
FLAT
BELLY
DIET
MEAL
}
Serve with ½ Open-Faced Spicy Salmon Sandwich (page 117), omitting the avocado (187).
TOTAL MEAL: 397 calories

Thai Crab and Sweet Corn Soup

■ PREP TIME: 15 MINUTES ■ TOTAL TIME: 30 MINUTES
■ MAKES 4 SERVINGS (1½ CUPS EACH) ■ MUFA: CANOLA OIL

Many, but not all, brands of fish sauce and soy sauce are gluten free. Be sure to carefully read labels when buying Asian sauces.

1 bag (16 ounces) frozen corn kernels, thawed, divided

3 cups gluten-free low-sodium vegetable broth, divided

¼ cup canola oil

1 red bell pepper, cut into thin strips

8 scallions, thinly sliced

1 jalapeño chile pepper, seeded and finely chopped (wear plastic gloves when handling)

1 tablespoon gluten-free reduced-sodium fish sauce

¾ pound fresh crabmeat, picked over to remove any cartilage or shells

¼ cup chopped fresh cilantro

¼ teaspoon ground red pepper

1. In a food processor, combine 1½ cups of the corn and 1½ cups of the broth. Pulse until smooth. Set aside.

2. In a large saucepan over medium-high heat, warm the oil. Add the bell pepper, scallions, and chile pepper and cook, stirring occasionally, for 6 minutes, or until tender.

3. Add the fish sauce, the reserved corn-broth mixture, the remaining corn kernels, and the remaining 1½ cups broth. Bring to a boil over medium-high heat. Reduce the heat to low, cover, and simmer for 10 minutes, or until thickened.

4. Stir in the crab, cilantro, and red pepper. Serve immediately.

Nutrition per serving: 357 calories, 24 g protein, 30 g carbohydrates, 16 g total fat, 1 g saturated fat, 5 g fiber, 658 mg sodium

Make It a FLAT BELLY DIET MEAL
Serve with ¼ cup shelled edamame (50).
TOTAL MEAL: 407 calories

Creamy Gazpacho

■ PREP TIME: 20 MINUTES ■ TOTAL TIME: 20 MINUTES + CHILLING TIME
■ SERVES 4 (1¼ CUPS EACH) ■ MUFA: PUMPKIN SEEDS

Thick and creamy Greek yogurt gives this cool summertime favorite a luscious texture.

2 large tomatoes (about 1 pound), cored and chopped

1½ cups 0% plain Greek yogurt

1 cup fresh cilantro leaves

¾ cup gluten-free mild or medium salsa

2 tablespoons sherry vinegar

1 teaspoon olive oil

2 cloves garlic, coarsely chopped

½ teaspoon salt

½ cup shelled unsalted roasted pumpkin seeds, divided

1. In a food processor, combine the tomatoes, yogurt, cilantro, salsa, vinegar, oil, garlic, salt, and ¼ cup of the pumpkin seeds. Pulse until smooth. Transfer the mixture to a large bowl. Cover and refrigerate for at least 2 hours, or until chilled.

2. Ladle into 4 bowls and top each with 1 tablespoon of the remaining pumpkin seeds.

Nutrition per serving: 176 calories, 13 g protein, 14 g carbohydrates, 9 g total fat, 1.5 g saturated fat, 2 g fiber, 527 mg sodium

Make It a FLAT BELLY DIET MEAL

Serve with ½ Grilled Cheese with Ham and Tomatoes (page 108) (213).
TOTAL MEAL: 389 calories

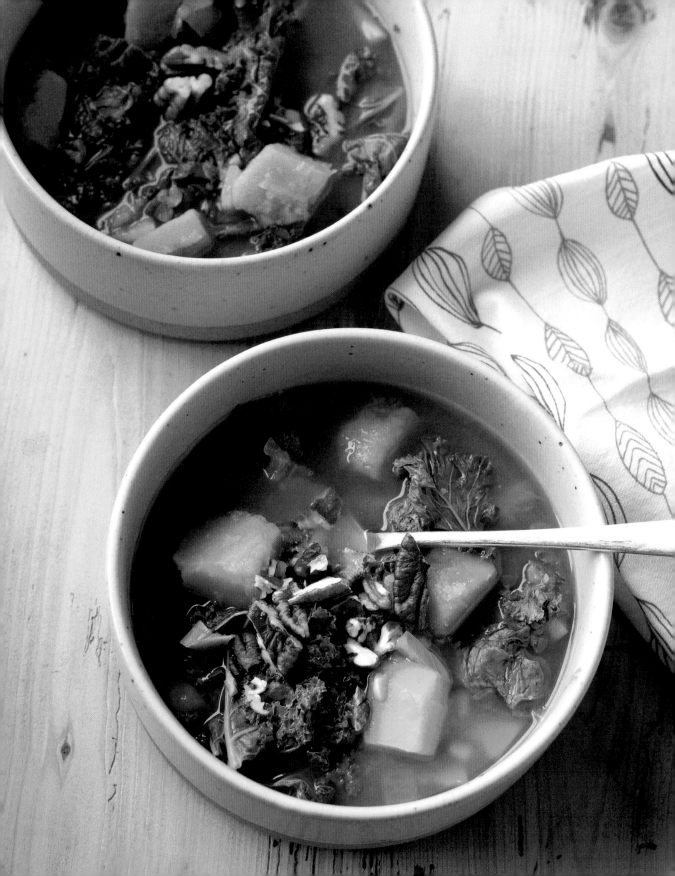

Butternut Squash and Kale
Soup with Pecans

▥ PREP TIME: 15 MINUTES ▥ TOTAL TIME: 30 MINUTES ▥ MAKES 4 SERVINGS (1¾ CUPS EACH)
▥ MUFA: PECANS

Squash and greens are a natural pairing, but the addition of toasted pecans raises this delicious soup to new levels. Any winter squash can be substituted for the butternut squash called for here.

1 teaspoon canola oil
1 onion, chopped
3 cloves garlic, minced
1 tablespoon grated fresh ginger
½ teaspoon salt
1 package (20 ounces) peeled butternut squash, cut into 1" pieces

4 cups gluten-free low-sodium vegetable broth
2 cups coarsely chopped kale
½ cup toasted chopped pecans
Gluten-free hot-pepper sauce (optional)

1. In a large nonstick saucepan over medium-high heat, warm the oil. Add the onion, garlic, ginger, and salt and cook, stirring frequently, for 2 to 3 minutes, or until fragrant.

2. Add the squash, broth, and kale and bring to a boil over high heat. Reduce the heat to low, cover, and simmer for 10 minutes, or until the squash is fork-tender. If desired, smash some pieces of the squash against the side of the pan to thicken the broth.

3. Ladle into 4 bowls and top each with 2 tablespoons of the pecans. Pass the hot-pepper sauce, if using, at the table.

Nutrition per serving: 216 calories, 4 g protein, 28 g carbohydrates, 11 g total fat, 1 g saturated fat, 6 g fiber, 452 mg sodium

Make It a
FLAT
BELLY
DIET
MEAL

Serve with a medium pear (104) sliced over ¼ cup fat-free ricotta cheese (50) and drizzled with 1 teaspoon honey (21).
TOTAL MEAL: 391 calories

Grilled Cheese with Ham and Tomatoes

■ PREP TIME: 5 MINUTES ■ TOTAL TIME: 10 MINUTES ■ MAKES 1 SERVING ■ MUFA: OLIVE OIL

To change it up, use equal amounts of smoked turkey and provolone cheese.

2 slices gluten-free multigrain bread

1 tablespoon olive oil

1 teaspoon gluten-free Dijon mustard

2 ounces thinly sliced gluten-free low-sodium deli ham

2 slices tomato

½ ounce thinly sliced reduced-fat Swiss cheese

¼ cup mixed greens

1. Lay the bread on a work surface and brush one side of both slices with the olive oil until all of the oil is absorbed. Flip 1 slice, oiled side down, and top with the mustard, ham, tomato, cheese, and greens. Top with the remaining slice of bread, oiled side up.

2. Coat a medium nonstick skillet with cooking spray and heat over medium-high heat. Cook the sandwich for 1 minute, pressing with a spatula, until browned on the bottom. Flip and cook for 1 minute, pressing lightly with the spatula, until browned on the second side. If the cheese is not quite melted, remove the pan from the heat, cover, and let sit for 30 seconds. Cut in half to serve.

Nutrition per serving: 375 calories, 19 g protein, 28 g carbohydrates, 22 g total fat, 3.5 g saturated fat, 2 g fiber, 891 mg sodium

Make It a
FLAT
BELLY
DIET
MEAL
} A single serving of this recipe counts as a Flat Belly Diet meal without any add-ons!

Ham and Black Olive Panini

■ PREP TIME: 5 MINUTES ■ TOTAL TIME: 10 MINUTES ■ MAKES 1 SERVING
■ MUFA: BLACK OLIVE TAPENADE

Be sure to use soft sun-dried tomatoes that are not packed in oil. They are moist, bright red, and require no soaking. Look for them in the produce section of your supermarket.

2 tablespoons Black Olive Tapenade (page 80) or store-bought gluten-free tapenade

2 slices gluten-free multigrain bread

1/4 cup arugula

2 ounces thinly sliced gluten-free low-sodium deli ham

1/2 ounce thinly sliced low-sodium muenster cheese

3 sun-dried tomatoes, cut into thin strips

1. Spread the tapenade on 1 slice of bread. Top with the arugula, ham, cheese, and sun-dried tomatoes. Top with the remaining slice of bread.

2. Coat a medium nonstick skillet with cooking spray and heat over medium-high heat, or heat a panini sandwich maker according to the manufacturer's instructions. Grill the sandwich for 4 minutes, turning once, or until the bread is well-marked and the cheese is melted. Cut in half to serve.

Nutrition per serving: 315 calories, 19 g protein, 30 g carbohydrates, 14 g total fat, 3 g saturated fat, 3 g fiber, 1,129 mg sodium

Make It a
FLAT
BELLY
DIET
MEAL

Serve with 2 cups salad greens drizzled with 2 tablespoons balsamic vinaigrette (98).
TOTAL MEAL: 413 calories

Smoky Avocado BLT

▦ PREP TIME: 20 MINUTES ▦ TOTAL TIME: 20 MINUTES ▦ MAKES 1 SERVING ▦ MUFA: AVOCADO

Chipotles in adobo sauce are smoked jalapeños in a spicy tomato sauce. They provide just the right amount of heat to this tasty sandwich. Store unused chipotle chiles in adobo sauce in an airtight container in the refrigerator for up to 1 month or in the freezer for up to 3 months.

¼ Hass avocado, peeled, pitted, and cubed

1 chipotle chile pepper in adobo sauce, chopped

1 teaspoon lime juice

1 slice gluten-free deli-style sourdough sandwich bread, toasted

2 leaves Boston lettuce

2 slices tomato

3 slices low-sodium crisp-cooked bacon

In a small bowl, mash the avocado, chile pepper, and lime juice until blended. Spread on the toast. Top with the lettuce, tomato, and bacon. Cut in half to serve.

Nutrition per serving: 302 calories, 9 g protein, 27 g carbohydrates, 16 g total fat, 4.5 g saturated fat, 6 g fiber, 651 mg sodium

Make It a FLAT BELLY DIET MEAL

Serve with 2 cups salad greens drizzled with 2 tablespoons balsamic vinaigrette (98).

TOTAL MEAL: 400 calories

Tangy Roast Beef Lettuce Wraps

■ PREP TIME: 15 MINUTES ■ TOTAL TIME: 15 MINUTES ■ MAKES 4 SERVINGS
■ MUFA: CANOLA OIL MAYONNAISE

If you prefer a milder flavor, omit the horseradish and add 1 tablespoon mango chutney to the mayonnaise instead.

¼ cup canola oil mayonnaise	1 apple, cut into 16 slices
2 teaspoons prepared horseradish, drained	4 slices (½ ounce each) low-fat Jarlsberg cheese
4 leaves green leaf lettuce	1 tomato, cut into 8 slices
4 slices (1½ ounces each) gluten-free low-sodium deli roast beef	

1. In a small bowl, combine the mayonnaise and horseradish until blended.

2. Place the lettuce leaves on a work surface. Spread each with one-fourth of the mayonnaise mixture. Evenly layer the roast beef, apple, cheese, and tomato down the center of each lettuce leaf. Fold each leaf around the filling and serve.

Nutrition per serving: 175 calories, 16 g protein, 9 g carbohydrates, 8 g total fat, 2 g saturated fat, 2 g fiber, 222 mg sodium

Make It a
FLAT
BELLY
DIET
MEAL
}
Serve with Cumin-Scented Kale Chips (page 238) (178) and ½ cup fresh pineapple chunks (41).
TOTAL MEAL: 394 calories

Roast Beef Panini

▓ PREP TIME: 10 MINUTES ▓ TOTAL TIME: 15 MINUTES ▓ MAKES 1 SERVING ▓ MUFA: AVOCADO

Pressed sandwiches like this panini taste great because of the many delicious flavors that meld during cooking.

2 slices gluten-free multigrain bread

2 ounces gluten-free store-roasted, deli-sliced lean roast beef

2 slices tomato

¼ Hass avocado, peeled, pitted, and sliced

¼ cup baby arugula

1 teaspoon gluten-free honey mustard

¼ teaspoon extra-virgin olive oil

1. Place 1 slice of bread on a work surface. Top with the roast beef, tomato, avocado, and arugula. Spread the remaining slice of bread with the mustard and set the slice, mustard side down, on the arugula.

2. Coat a medium nonstick skillet with the oil and heat over medium heat. Lightly coat both sides of the sandwich with cooking spray and place in the pan. Place a heavy pan on top of the sandwich. Cook for 2 minutes, or until lightly browned. Flip and cook for 2 minutes, or until lightly browned and warm in the center. Cut in half to serve.

Nutrition per serving: 369 calories, 18 g protein, 42 g carbohydrates, 17 g total fat, 2 g saturated fat, 8 g fiber, 407 mg sodium

Make It a FLAT BELLY DIET MEAL

Serve with ½ cup sliced mango (53).
TOTAL MEAL: 422 calories

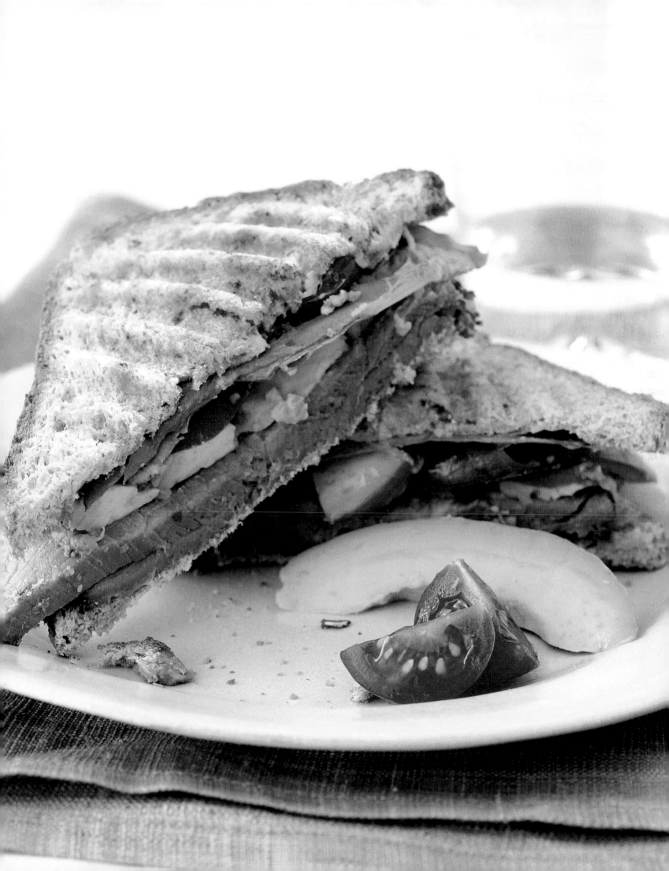

Tuna Melt

▦ PREP TIME: 10 MINUTES ▦ TOTAL TIME: 15 MINUTES ▦ MAKES 2 SERVINGS
▦ MUFA: CANOLA OIL MAYONNAISE

Peppery arugula leaves add bite to this American favorite.

1 can (5 ounces) reduced-sodium water-packed tuna, drained and flaked

2 tablespoons canola oil mayonnaise

1 rib celery, finely chopped

1 tablespoon finely chopped red onion

1 teaspoon lemon juice

2 slices gluten-free multigrain bread

¼ cup baby arugula

4 slices tomato

2 slices (½ ounce each) part-skim mozzarella cheese

⅛ teaspoon salt

1. In a medium bowl, combine the tuna, mayonnaise, celery, onion, and lemon juice until well mixed.

2. Preheat the broiler.

3. Place the bread slices on a work surface. Top each slice with half of the arugula, tuna mixture, tomato, and cheese. Place the sandwiches on the broiler-pan rack and broil 4″ from the heat for 2 minutes, or until the cheese is melted.

Nutrition per serving: 239 calories, 20 g protein, 15 g carbohydrates, 11 g total fat, 2 g saturated fat, 1 g fiber, 377 mg sodium

**Make It a
FLAT
BELLY
DIET
MEAL**
Serve with ¾ cup fresh orange juice (84) and 1 cup red or green grapes (104).
TOTAL MEAL: 427 calories

Mediterranean Salmon Salad Sandwiches

■ PREP TIME: 5 MINUTES ■ TOTAL TIME: 5 MINUTES ■ MAKES 2 SERVINGS
■ MUFA: BLACK OLIVE TAPENADE

These open-faced sandwiches are packed with essential omega-3 fatty acids. The tapenade packs a flavorful MUFA punch!

1 can (5 ounces) pink salmon, drained

1 medium tomato, chopped

¼ cup crumbled reduced-fat goat cheese

1 tablespoon lemon juice

¼ cup Black Olive Tapenade (page 80) or store-bought gluten-free tapenade

2 slices gluten-free flax bread, toasted

1. In a medium bowl, combine the salmon, tomato, goat cheese, and lemon juice until blended.

2. Spread the tapenade over both slices of toast and top each with half of the salmon mixture. Cut each in half to serve.

Nutrition per serving: 235 calories, 18 g protein, 17 g carbohydrates, 12 g total fat, 2 g saturated fat, 5 g fiber, 624 mg sodium

Make It a
FLAT
BELLY
DIET
MEAL

Serve with a Berry-Avocado Smoothie (page 248), omitting the avocado (127), and a salad made from ½ sliced cucumber (12) tossed with 1 cup grape tomatoes (30) and 2 tablespoons minced red onion (12). **TOTAL MEAL: 416 calories**

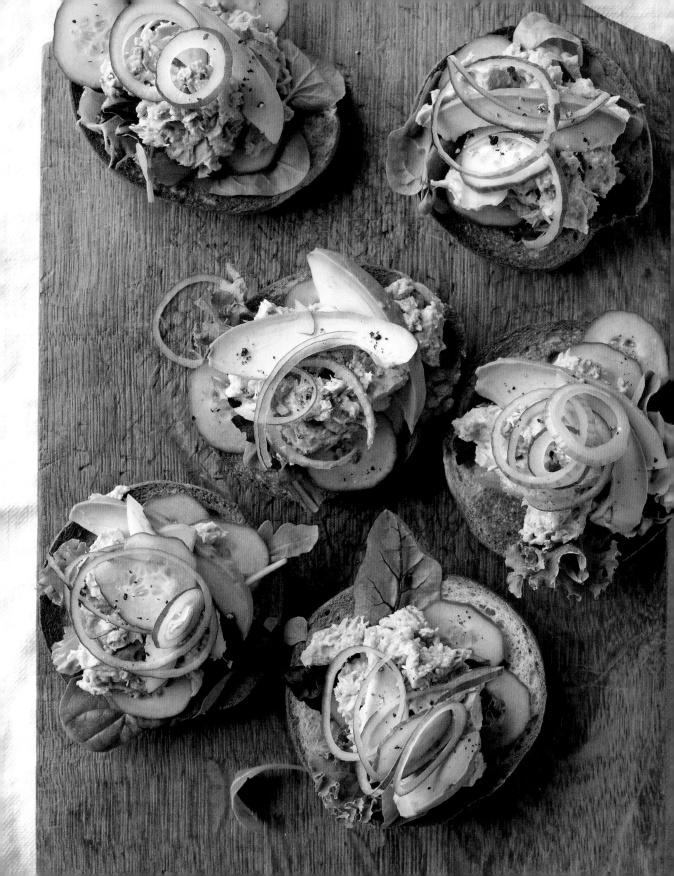

Open-Faced Spicy Salmon Sandwiches

PREP TIME: 15 MINUTES ▪ TOTAL TIME: 15 MINUTES ▪ MAKES 4 SERVINGS ▪ MUFA: AVOCADO

This is a great way to use leftover grilled salmon—you'll need about 2 cups coarsely mashed.

- 1 can (14.75 ounces) pink salmon, drained
- ¼ cup gluten-free reduced-fat horseradish-Dijon mayonnaise
- 2 gluten-free multigrain bagels, split and toasted
- 1 cup mixed baby greens
- 1 Hass avocado, peeled, pitted, and sliced
- ¼ small hothouse (seedless) cucumber, thinly sliced
- ¼ small red onion, thinly sliced

1. In a medium bowl, combine the salmon and mayonnaise, mashing with a fork until well mixed.

2. Place 4 bagel halves on a work surface. Top each half with one-fourth of the greens, salmon mixture, avocado, cucumber, and onion.

Nutrition per serving: 431 calories, 24 g protein, 42 g carbohydrates, 19 g total fat, 3 g saturated fat, 5 g fiber, 768 mg sodium

Make It a
FLAT
BELLY
DIET
MEAL

A single serving of this recipe counts as a Flat Belly Diet meal without any add-ons!

Tzatziki Chicken Wrap

■ PREP TIME: 15 MINUTES ■ TOTAL TIME: 15 MINUTES ■ MAKES 2 SERVINGS ■ MUFA: OLIVES

If you prefer a vegetarian version of this hearty wrap, substitute ½ cup cubed tofu in place of the chicken.

¼ small hothouse (seedless) cucumber, peeled and grated	2 gluten-free brown rice tortillas (8" diameter)
2 tablespoons 0% plain Greek yogurt	1 cup loosely packed baby spinach
20 kalamata olives, pitted and chopped	4 ounces thinly sliced gluten-free low-sodium deli chicken breast
1 tablespoon chopped fresh dill	4 slices tomato
1 teaspoon lemon juice	

1. In a small bowl, combine the cucumber, yogurt, olives, dill, and lemon juice until well mixed.

2. Transfer the tortillas to a work surface. Spread half of the tzatziki over each tortilla. Layer each with half of the spinach, chicken, and tomato down the center. Fold the short sides over the filling, then roll up burrito style to enclose the filling. Cut each wrap in half and serve at once.

Nutrition per serving: 323 calories, 18 g protein, 33 g carbohydrates, 14 g total fat, 1 g saturated fat, 4 g fiber, 1,154 mg sodium

Make It a FLAT BELLY DIET MEAL

Serve with 2 cups chopped watermelon (80).
TOTAL MEAL: 403 calories

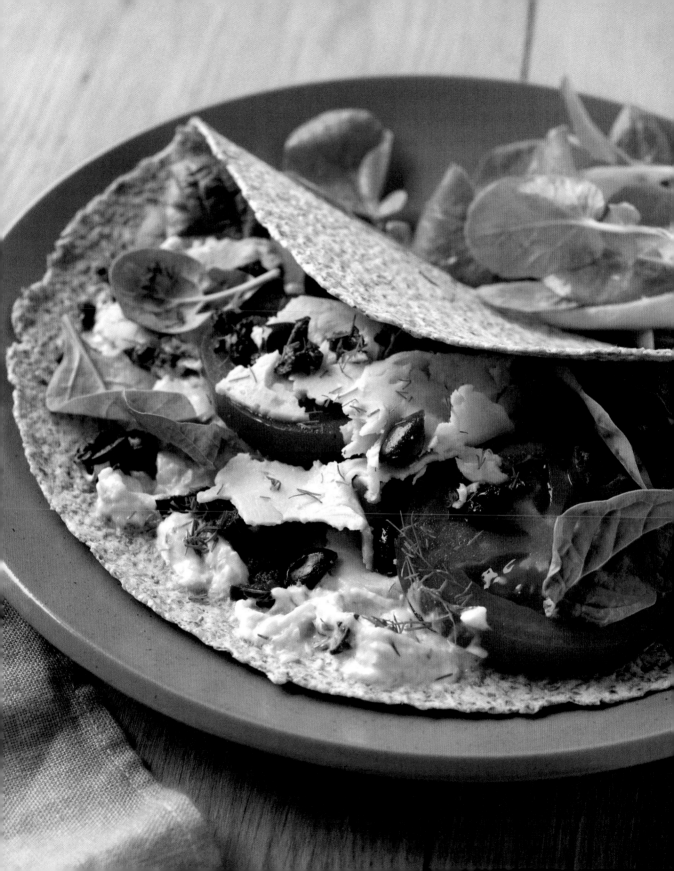

Cheesy Chicken Tostada

■ PREP TIME: 10 MINUTES ■ TOTAL TIME: 15 MINUTES ■ MAKES 2 SERVINGS ■ MUFA: CANOLA OIL

This is a snap to put together when using leftover chicken. But you can use any protein you have on hand—try it with strips of grilled steak or fish, or even canned black beans or pieces of tofu.

2 tablespoons canola oil

2 gluten-free corn tortillas

2 slices (½ ounce each) reduced-fat pepper Jack cheese

1 cup cooked shredded chicken breast

½ cup shredded romaine lettuce

2 tablespoons gluten-free salsa

2 tablespoons chopped fresh cilantro

1. In a large nonstick skillet over medium-high heat, warm the oil. Cook the tortillas for about 1 minute on each side, or until lightly browned (they will become crisp as they cool). Transfer the tortillas to a work surface.

2. Place the tortillas on each of 2 plates. Top each with half of the cheese, chicken, lettuce, salsa, and cilantro. Serve at once.

Nutrition per serving: 344 calories, 28 g protein, 12 g carbohydrates, 20 g total fat, 4 g saturated fat, 2 g fiber, 261 mg sodium

Make It a FLAT BELLY DIET MEAL

Serve with 2 tablespoons reduced-fat sour cream (40).
TOTAL MEAL: 384 calories

Turkey MUFAletta Wrap

▧ PREP TIME: 10 MINUTES ▧ TOTAL TIME: 10 MINUTES ▧ MAKES 2 SERVINGS ▧ MUFA: OLIVES

Taste how an ordinary turkey sandwich becomes extraordinary with a hearty topping of spicy olive salad. When using olives, it's important to watch the sodium content of your other ingredients. Boar's Head and Applegate Farms are two good sources for lower-sodium turkey breast.

10 green pimiento-stuffed olives, pitted and chopped

10 black olives, pitted and chopped

1 teaspoon balsamic vinegar

⅛ teaspoon red-pepper flakes

2 gluten-free brown rice tortillas (8″ diameter)

4 ounces thinly sliced gluten-free low-sodium deli turkey breast

1 slice (½ ounce) reduced-fat low-sodium provolone cheese

½ cup mixed baby greens

1. In a small bowl, combine the green and black olives, vinegar, and red-pepper flakes until well mixed.

2. Place the tortillas on a work surface. Layer each with half of the turkey, cheese, greens, and olive mixture down the center. Fold the short sides over the filling, then roll up burrito style to enclose the filling. Cut each wrap in half and serve at once.

Nutrition per serving: 297 calories, 16 g protein, 28 g carbohydrates, 12 g total fat, 1 g saturated fat, 2 g fiber, 1,132 mg sodium

Make It a
FLAT
BELLY
DIET
MEAL

Serve with 2 cups salad greens with 2 tablespoons balsamic vinaigrette (98).
TOTAL MEAL: 395 calories

SALADS

Steak Salad with Creamy Avocado Dressing

■ PREP TIME: 15 MINUTES ■ TOTAL TIME: 35 MINUTES ■ MAKES 4 SERVINGS ■ MUFA: AVOCADO

The avocado dressing is also wonderful served alongside crunchy dippers like carrots, bell peppers, and cucumbers.

¾ pound sirloin steak, trimmed of all visible fat

½ teaspoon salt, divided

1 Hass avocado, peeled, pitted, and chopped

½ cup 0% plain Greek yogurt

¼ cup lime juice

½ teaspoon ground cumin

6 cups mixed baby greens

1 cup cherry tomatoes, halved

1 cup canned black beans, rinsed and drained

¼ cup chopped fresh cilantro

1. Sprinkle the steak with ¼ teaspoon of the salt. Heat a large nonstick skillet coated with cooking spray over medium-high heat. Cook the steak for 8 to 10 minutes for medium-rare or to the desired doneness, turning once. Transfer the steak to a cutting board and let stand 10 minutes before thinly slicing.

2. Meanwhile, in a food processor, combine the avocado, yogurt, lime juice, cumin, and the remaining ¼ teaspoon salt. Process until smooth.

3. In a large bowl, combine the greens, tomatoes, beans, and cilantro. Toss with the avocado dressing until well coated.

4. Divide the salad among 4 plates and top evenly with one-fourth of the steak.

Nutrition per serving: 279 calories, 26 g protein, 18 g carbohydrates, 12 g total fat, 2.5 g saturated fat, 7 g fiber, 575 mg sodium

Make It a FLAT BELLY DIET MEAL

Serve with ½ cup gluten-free penne pasta (106) topped with ¼ cup gluten-free tomato sauce (15).
TOTAL MEAL: 400 calories

Shrimp and Avocado Salad with Ranch Dressing

■ PREP TIME: 20 MINUTES ■ TOTAL TIME: 20 MINUTES ■ MAKES 4 SERVINGS ■ MUFA: AVOCADO

This salad is just as delicious made with grilled salmon or leftover chicken.

¼ cup mayonnaise

¼ cup buttermilk

1 tablespoon chopped fresh tarragon

2 teaspoons gluten-free Dijon mustard

2 teaspoons lemon juice

¾ pound small cooked peeled and deveined shrimp

1 Hass avocado, peeled, pitted, and cubed

1 cup cherry tomatoes, halved

2 ribs celery, finely chopped

2 cups mixed baby greens

1. In a large bowl, whisk together the mayonnaise, buttermilk, tarragon, mustard, and lemon juice. Add the shrimp, avocado, tomatoes, and celery and toss gently to coat.

2. Divide the greens evenly among 4 plates. Top with the shrimp mixture and serve at once.

Nutrition per serving: 217 calories, 23 g protein, 10 g carbohydrates, 10 g total fat, 1 g saturated fat, 4 g fiber, 421 mg sodium

Make It a FLAT BELLY DIET MEAL

Serve with Caramelized Onion and Olive Focaccia (page 252), omitting the olives (166).
TOTAL MEAL: 383 calories

Orange, Apple, and Jicama Slaw with Scallops

■ PREP TIME: 15 MINUTES ■ TOTAL TIME: 20 MINUTES ■ MAKES 4 SERVINGS
■ MUFA: PUMPKIN SEEDS

When working with jicama, make sure to wash and peel it just before using because, like potatoes and avocados, the flesh will darken when exposed to air.

3 tablespoons lime juice

3 tablespoons chopped fresh cilantro

2 teaspoons sugar

½ teaspoon salt, divided

1 jicama, peeled and cut into thin strips

1 large apple, peeled, cored, and cut into thin matchsticks

1 orange, peeled and cut into sections

½ cup shelled unsalted dry-roasted pumpkin seeds

1 teaspoon olive oil

¾ pound sea scallops

1. In a large bowl, whisk together the lime juice, cilantro, sugar, and ¼ teaspoon of the salt. Add the jicama, apple, orange, and pumpkin seeds. Toss well.

2. In a large nonstick skillet over medium-high heat, warm the oil. Sprinkle the scallops with the remaining ¼ teaspoon salt and add to the skillet. Cook for 2 to 3 minutes per side, or until opaque.

3. Serve the slaw topped with the scallops.

Nutrition per serving: 291 calories, 20 g protein, 34 g carbohydrates, 9 g total fat, 1.5 g saturated fat, 11 g fiber, 437 mg sodium

Make It a FLAT BELLY DIET MEAL

Serve with ½ cup Creamy Southern-Style Peanut Soup (page 102) (110).
TOTAL MEAL: 401 calories

Tuna Mac Salad

■ PREP TIME: 5 MINUTES ■ TOTAL TIME: 15 MINUTES ■ MAKES 4 SERVINGS
■ MUFA: CANOLA OIL MAYONNAISE

White tuna is loaded with valuable omega-3s, a type of fat that helps reduce inflammation. But if you're concerned about mercury levels found in seafood, opt for canned salmon or light tuna (versus white tuna) in this recipe.

6 ounces gluten-free brown rice elbow or other small shell pasta

2 cans (5 ounces each) no-salt-added water-packed solid white tuna, drained

1 red bell pepper, cut into thin strips

2 carrots, thinly sliced

2 ribs celery, thinly sliced

½ red onion, finely chopped

¼ cup canola oil mayonnaise

¼ cup chopped fresh parsley

¼ teaspoon salt

¼ teaspoon ground black pepper

1. Bring a large pot of water to a boil. Add the pasta and cook according to package directions. Drain, rinse under cold water, and drain again. Transfer to a large bowl.

2. Add the tuna, bell pepper, carrots, celery, onion, mayonnaise, parsley, salt, and black pepper. Toss to mix well.

Nutrition per serving: 308 calories, 18 g protein, 41 g carbohydrates, 8 g total fat, 1 g saturated fat, 4 g fiber, 355 mg sodium

Make It a FLAT BELLY DIET MEAL

Serve with 2 slices toasted gluten-free rice bread (100).
TOTAL MEAL: 408 calories

Tuscan Tuna and White Bean Salad

■ PREP TIME: 10 MINUTES ■ TOTAL TIME: 10 MINUTES ■ MAKES 4 SERVINGS ■ MUFA: OLIVE OIL

A classic pairing with just a few pantry ingredients, cannellini beans and canned tuna make a satisfying lunch or a quick weeknight dinner.

¼ cup olive oil

2 teaspoons grated lemon peel

3 tablespoons lemon juice

1 tablespoon gluten-free stone-ground mustard

¼ teaspoon salt

6 cups torn escarole

2 cans (5 ounces each) no-salt-added water-packed chunk light tuna, drained

1 can (15½ ounces) cannellini beans, rinsed and drained

1 large tomato, chopped

½ small red onion, finely chopped

½ cup chopped fresh basil

1. In a large bowl, whisk together the olive oil, lemon peel, lemon juice, mustard, and salt.

2. Add the escarole, tuna, beans, tomato, onion, and basil, tossing gently to mix well. Serve at once.

Nutrition per serving: 288 calories, 20 g protein, 18 g carbohydrates, 16 g total fat, 2.5 g saturated fat, 7 g fiber, 438 mg sodium

Make It a FLAT BELLY DIET MEAL

Serve with 1 toasted gluten-free English muffin (130).
TOTAL MEAL: 418 calories

Cauliflower, Tomato, and Pesto Pasta Salad

▓ PREP TIME: 10 MINUTES ▓ TOTAL TIME: 20 MINUTES ▓ MAKES 4 SERVINGS ▓ MUFA: PESTO

At the peak of summer, using the same water to cook both pasta and a vegetable is a good way to stay cool. As a bonus, it cuts down a pot to clean! For best results, make this dish early in the day to allow time for the flavors to blend.

4 ounces gluten-free brown rice rotini pasta

2 cups cauliflower florets

1 cup grape tomatoes, halved

¼ red onion, thinly sliced

¼ cup chopped fresh basil

¼ cup Pesto (page 84) or store-bought gluten-free pesto

1. Prepare the pasta according to package directions, adding the cauliflower during the last 2 minutes of cooking time. Drain. Rinse under cold running water, then drain again. Transfer to a large bowl.

2. Add the tomatoes, onion, and basil to the bowl with the pasta. Stir in the pesto and toss to coat well. Refrigerate until ready to serve.

Nutrition per serving: 182 calories, 5 g protein, 27 g carbohydrates, 7 g total fat, 1 g saturated fat, 3 g fiber, 117 mg sodium

Make It a FLAT BELLY DIET MEAL

Serve with 3 ounces roasted chicken breast (140) and ½ cup grilled baby red potatoes (75).
TOTAL MEAL: 397 calories

Crunchy Garden Salad with Green Goddess Dressing

■ PREP TIME: 15 MINUTES ■ TOTAL TIME: 15 MINUTES ■ MAKES 4 SERVINGS
■ MUFA: CANOLA OIL MAYONNAISE

This dressing, invented in the 1920s, is a California classic. Our version is a little lighter than the original, but every bit as delicious. Top with our Parmesan-Pepper Croutons, if you like.

½ cup 2% plain Greek yogurt
¼ cup canola oil mayonnaise
¼ cup chopped fresh parsley
2 scallions, chopped
1 tablespoon white wine vinegar
1 tablespoon chopped fresh tarragon
1 clove garlic, minced
Pinch of salt

1 container (7 ounces) mixed baby greens
1 cup grape tomatoes, halved
1 cup baby carrots
½ hothouse (seedless) cucumber, halved lengthwise and cut crosswise into half moons
¼ cup sliced radishes
¼ cup Parmesan-Pepper Croutons (optional)

1. In a food processor, combine the yogurt, mayonnaise, parsley, scallions, vinegar, tarragon, garlic, and salt. Pulse until smooth.

2. In a large bowl, combine the greens, tomatoes, carrots, cucumber, and radishes. Add the dressing and toss to coat well. Top with the croutons, if using.

Nutrition per serving: 160 calories, 5 g protein, 10 g carbohydrates, 12 g total fat, 1 g saturated fat, 3 g fiber, 208 mg sodium

Make It a FLAT BELLY DIET MEAL
Serve with 4 ounces thinly sliced broiled flank steak (218) and 1 cup steamed asparagus (40).
TOTAL MEAL: 418 calories

PARMESAN-PEPPER CROUTONS

Homemade croutons are easy to make. Cut 2 slices (1½ ounces each) gluten-free 7-grain sandwich bread into ¾" cubes. In a medium nonstick skillet over medium heat, warm 1 tablespoon olive oil. Toast the bread cubes for 2 to 3 minutes, shaking the pan occasionally, or until golden brown. Transfer the croutons to a medium bowl and toss with 2 teaspoons grated Parmesan cheese, ¼ teaspoon ground black pepper, and a pinch of coarse salt. Makes 1 cup. One serving (¼ cup croutons) adds 9 calories, 1 g protein, 14 g carbohydrates, 5 g total fat, 0.5 g saturated fat, 2 g fiber, and 160 mg sodium to your meal.

Tropical Turkey Salad

▥ PREP TIME: 15 MINUTES ▥ TOTAL TIME: 30 MINUTES ▥ MAKES 4 SERVINGS ▥ MUFA: AVOCADO

Jerk seasoning, traditionally used in Jamaican cooking, is a flavorful blend of allspice, thyme, garlic, onion, and habanero chile pepper. If you're concerned about spiciness, no worries—the sweetness of this citrus salad balances the heat.

1 tablespoon gluten-free low-sodium jerk seasoning

3 tablespoons lime juice, divided

1 teaspoon + 2 tablespoons olive oil

4 boneless, skinless turkey cutlets (4 ounces each)

1 tablespoon orange juice

½ teaspoon honey

¼ teaspoon salt

6 cups colorful mixed greens

¼ small white onion, thinly sliced

1 mango, peeled, pitted, and sliced

1 Hass avocado, peeled, pitted, and sliced

1. In a small bowl, mix together the jerk seasoning, 1 tablespoon of the lime juice, and 1 teaspoon oil until blended. Rub on both sides of the cutlets.

2. Coat a nonstick ridged grill pan with cooking spray and set over medium-high heat. Cook the cutlets for 8 minutes, turning once, or until no longer pink and the juices run clear. Transfer to a plate. Let stand for 5 minutes before slicing into thin slices.

3. In a large bowl, whisk together the orange juice, honey, salt, the remaining 2 tablespoons lime juice, and 2 tablespoons oil. Add the greens and onion and toss to coat. Add the mango and avocado and gently toss.

4. Divide the salad among 4 plates and top each with one-fourth of the turkey.

Nutrition per serving: 309 calories, 30 g protein, 17 g carbohydrates, 14 g total fat, 2 g saturated fat, 5 g fiber, 271 mg sodium

Make It a
FLAT
BELLY
DIET
MEAL

Serve with ½ serving of Garlic Tostones (page 239) (118).
TOTAL MEAL: 427 calories

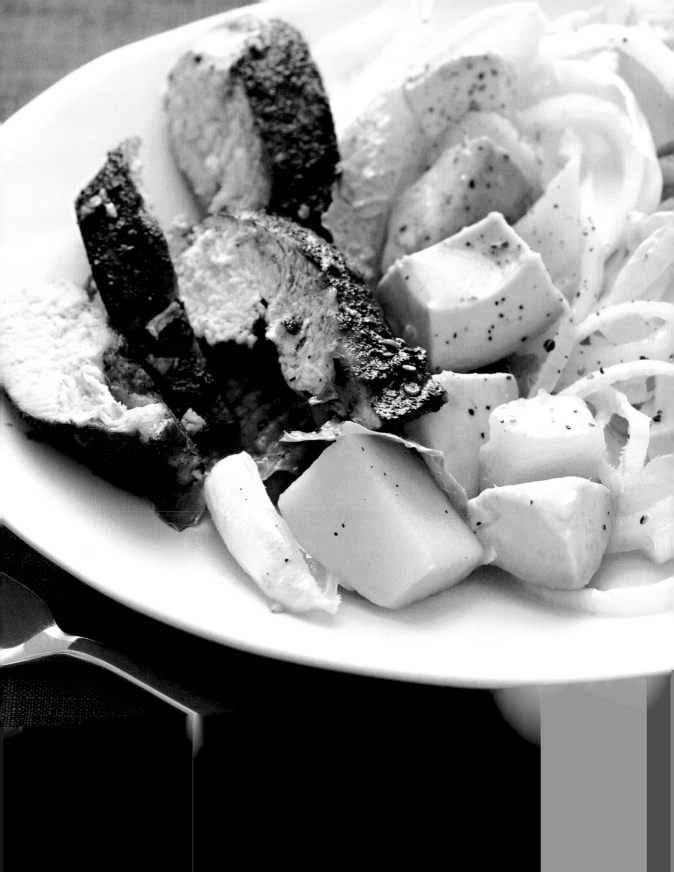

Roast Chicken and Fresh Corn Salad

■ PREP TIME: 15 MINUTES ■ TOTAL TIME: 15 MINUTES ■ MAKES 4 SERVINGS
■ MUFA: OLIVES, OLIVE OIL

Here's a delicious way to use fresh corn when it's in season. One ear of fresh corn will yield about ½ cup of kernels.

2 cups roasted chicken breast, cut into ½" pieces

2 large ears corn, shucked (about 1 cup)

1 red bell pepper, chopped

1 small red onion, thinly sliced

10 oil-cured black olives, pitted and chopped

10 kalamata olives, pitted and chopped

2 tablespoons lime juice

2 tablespoons olive oil

¼ teaspoon salt

In a large bowl, combine the chicken, corn, bell pepper, onion, olives, lime juice, olive oil, and salt. Toss to coat well. Serve at once.

Nutrition per serving: 291 calories, 25 g protein, 19 g carbohydrates, 14 g total fat, 2 g saturated fat, 2 g fiber, 435 mg sodium

Make It a FLAT BELLY DIET MEAL

Serve with 2 cups chopped watermelon (80) and ½ cup red or green grapes (52).
TOTAL MEAL: 423 calories

Quinoa with Roasted Tomatoes, Walnuts, and Olives

■ PREP TIME: 10 MINUTES ■ TOTAL TIME: 30 MINUTES ■ MAKES 4 SERVINGS ■ MUFA: WALNUTS

Roasting brings out a candylike sweetness of the tomatoes, which nicely counters the bitter saltiness of the olives.

1 cup red quinoa

2 cups cherry tomatoes

10 oil-cured black olives, pitted

1 shallot, sliced

1 tablespoon chopped fresh rosemary

2 cloves garlic, sliced

2 tablespoons olive oil, divided

1 cup chopped fresh basil

½ cup toasted walnuts, coarsely chopped

1 tablespoon sherry vinegar

1. In a medium saucepan, bring 2 cups water to a boil over high heat. Add the quinoa and reduce to a simmer. Cover and cook for 20 minutes, or just until tender. Drain any remaining liquid and cool.

2. Meanwhile, preheat the oven to 425°F. On a small rimmed baking sheet or shallow roasting pan, combine the tomatoes, olives, shallot, rosemary, garlic, and 1 tablespoon of the oil. Toss to coat well. Roast for 20 minutes, stirring occasionally, or until the tomatoes are tender and lightly browned.

3. In a large bowl, combine the roasted tomato mixture, basil, walnuts, vinegar, and the remaining 1 tablespoon oil. Add the cooled quinoa and stir to combine well. Serve at room temperature.

Nutrition per serving: 357 calories, 10 g protein, 43 g carbohydrates, 19 g total fat, 2 g saturated fat, 7 g fiber, 82 mg sodium

Make It a FLAT BELLY DIET MEAL

Serve with 1 cup steamed broccoli (44).
TOTAL MEAL: 401 calories

Mango Millet Salad
with Orange-Sesame Dressing

▥ PREP TIME: 15 MINUTES ▥ TOTAL TIME: 45 MINUTES ▥ MAKES 4 SERVINGS ▥ MUFA: CASHEWS

Turn this nutrient-rich dish into a main-dish salad by topping it with grilled shrimp or chicken.

½ cup millet	1 teaspoon honey
1½ cups water	1 teaspoon toasted sesame oil
¼ cup orange juice	1 mango, peeled, pitted, and cubed
2 tablespoons cider vinegar	1 red bell pepper, chopped
2 teaspoons gluten-free reduced-sodium soy sauce	¼ cup chopped fresh cilantro
	½ cup chopped unsalted cashews

1. In a medium saucepan over medium-high heat, toast the millet, stirring constantly, for 2 to 3 minutes, or until the millet is fragrant and just begins to pop. Add the water and bring to a boil. Reduce the heat to low, cover, and simmer for 25 minutes, or until the millet is tender and any liquid is absorbed. Fluff with a fork and let cool.

2. Meanwhile, in a large bowl, whisk together the orange juice, vinegar, soy sauce, honey, and sesame oil. Add the mango, bell pepper, cilantro, cashews, and cooled millet. Toss to coat well. Serve chilled or at room temperature.

Nutrition per serving: 258 calories, 7 g protein, 37 g carbohydrates, 10 g total fat, 2 g saturated fat, 4 g fiber, 114 mg sodium

**Make It a
FLAT
BELLY
DIET
MEAL**

Serve with 3 ounces roasted pork tenderloin (122).
TOTAL MEAL: 380 calories

Spiced Lentil and Chickpea Salad with Tahini Dressing

▓ PREP TIME: 15 MINUTES ▓ TOTAL TIME: 35 MINUTES ▓ MAKES 4 SERVINGS
▓ MUFA: TAHINI, OLIVE OIL

Be sure to rinse the lentils and pick out any stones before using.

3/4 cup lentils

4 tablespoons tahini

1/4 cup warm water

2 tablespoons lemon juice

2 tablespoons olive oil

1/2 teaspoon ground cumin

1/4 teaspoon salt

1 can (14 ounces) chickpeas, rinsed and drained

1/4 hothouse (seedless) cucumber, chopped (about 1 cup)

1 tomato, chopped

1 cup chopped watercress

1. In a large saucepan, bring 4 cups water to a boil over high heat. Add the lentils and reduce to a simmer. Cover and cook for 20 minutes, or just until tender. Drain well and cool.

2. Meanwhile, in a large bowl, whisk together the tahini, warm water, lemon juice, olive oil, cumin, and salt until blended.

3. Add the chickpeas, cucumber, tomato, watercress, and the cooled lentils. Toss to coat well. Serve chilled or at room temperature.

Nutrition per serving: 365 calories, 16 g protein, 42 g carbohydrates, 16 g total fat, 2 g saturated fat, 16 g fiber, 364 mg sodium

Make It a FLAT BELLY DIET MEAL

Serve with 1 cup sliced strawberries (47).
TOTAL MEAL: 412 calories

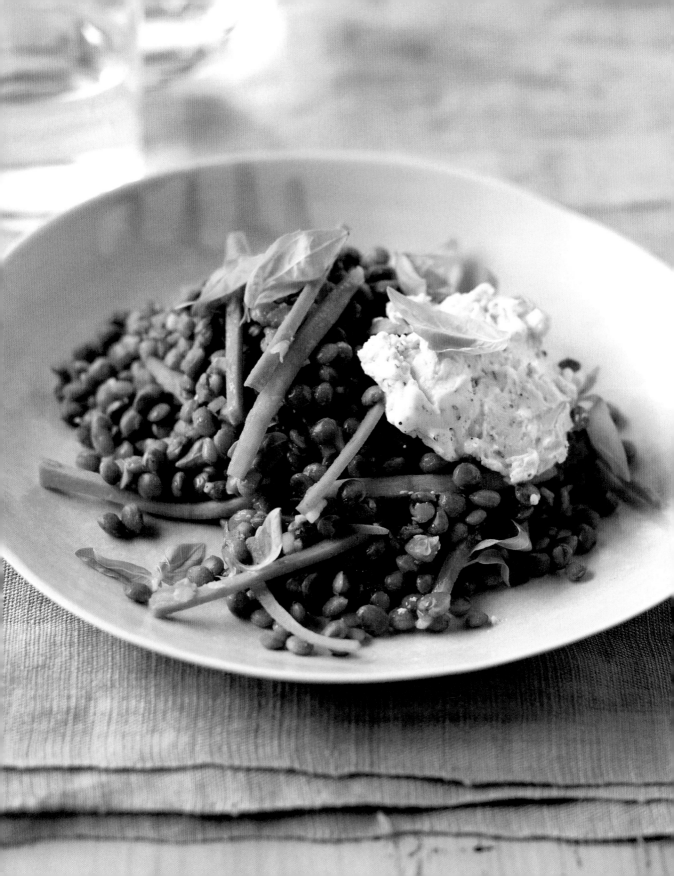

Lentil Salad with Basil and Goat Cheese

■ PREP TIME: 10 MINUTES ■ TOTAL TIME: 30 MINUTES ■ MAKES 4 SERVINGS ■ MUFA: WALNUT OIL

French lentils offer a subtle peppery flavor and tend to hold their shape better than regular brown lentils. They're often available in natural food stores that carry a variety of bulk ingredients. Of course, if necessary, regular brown lentils are a worthy stand-in in this easy salad.

1 cup French lentils	¼ teaspoon ground black pepper
¼ cup walnut oil	1 carrot, grated
2 tablespoons red wine vinegar	2 tablespoons chopped fresh basil
2 cloves garlic, minced	4 ounces gluten-free herbed goat cheese
¼ teaspoon salt	

1. In a large saucepan, bring 4 cups water to a boil over high heat. Add the lentils and reduce to a simmer. Cover and cook for 20 minutes, or just until tender. Drain well and cool.

2. In a large bowl, whisk together the oil, vinegar, garlic, salt, and pepper. Add the lentils, carrot, and basil. Toss to coat well.

3. Cut the goat cheese crosswise into four ¾"- thick rounds. Place on a small microwaveable plate. Cover and microwave on medium power for 30 seconds, or just until the cheese is warm.

4. Divide the lentil mixture among 4 plates. Place 1 cheese round on each plate and serve at once.

Nutrition per serving: 383 calories, 17 g protein, 30 g carbohydrates, 22 g total fat, 7 g saturated fat, 8 g fiber, 317 mg sodium

Make It a FLAT BELLY DIET MEAL A single serving of this recipe counts as a Flat Belly Diet Meal without any add-ons!

Indonesian Vegetable Salad

■ PREP TIME: 15 MINUTES ■ TOTAL TIME: 25 MINUTES ■ MAKES 4 SERVINGS ■ MUFA: PEANUT BUTTER

This colorful platter of fresh veggies uses store-bought peanut sauce and water—how simple is that? And you can add a dash of hot sauce if the mood strikes.

2 cups green beans, trimmed

2 carrots, thinly sliced

2 cups mixed baby greens

1 red bell pepper, cut into ¾" pieces

½ hothouse (seedless) cucumber, thinly sliced

1 hard-cooked egg, peeled and chopped

1 cup loosely packed cilantro leaves

1 cup peanut sauce (see below) or store-bought sodium-free gluten-free prepared peanut sauce

3–4 tablespoons water

1. Bring a large pot of water to a boil over high heat. Add the green beans and carrots, reduce the heat to medium, cover, and simmer for 5 minutes, or until tender-crisp. Drain and rinse under cold running water and drain again.

2. Arrange the baby greens on a large platter. Top with the green beans, carrots, bell pepper, and cucumber. Top with the chopped egg and sprinkle with cilantro.

3. Whisk together the peanut sauce and enough water in a small bowl to make a smooth, pourable consistency. Drizzle the sauce over the vegetables and serve at once.

Nutrition per serving: 168 calories, 4 g protein, 22 g carbohydrates, 6 g total fat, 0.5 g saturated fat, 4 g fiber, 50 mg sodium

Make It a FLAT BELLY DIET MEAL Serve with 3 ounces roasted chicken breast, cut into strips (140), and ½ cup cooked quinoa (111).
TOTAL MEAL: 419 calories

MAKE YOUR OWN PEANUT SAUCE

In a small saucepan over medium heat, combine 1 cup chunky natural unsalted peanut butter, ¾ cup gluten-free, reduced-sodium chicken broth, ⅓ cup light unsweetened coconut milk, 3 tablespoons packed brown sugar, 2 tablespoons freshly squeezed lime juice, 1 tablespoon gluten-free, low-sodium fish sauce, 1 tablespoon grated peeled fresh ginger, and ⅛ teaspoon red-pepper flakes. Cook, stirring often, for 2 to 3 minutes or until very smooth and slightly thickened.

Carrot-Raisin Salad
with Pickled Ginger Dressing

▦ PREP TIME: 15 MINUTES ▦ TOTAL TIME: 25 MINUTES ▦ MAKES 4 SERVINGS ▦ MUFA: WALNUTS

Instead of the traditional mayonnaise-based dressing, this classic has been updated with a light pickled ginger dressing. Pickled ginger is thinly sliced fresh ginger preserved in seasoned rice vinegar. It is sold in jars and can be found in the Asian aisle of your supermarket.

⅓ cup golden raisins	⅛ teaspoon salt
1 tablespoon gluten-free rice vinegar	2 cups grated carrots
1 tablespoon pickled ginger, finely chopped + 1 tablespoon pickled ginger juice	½ cup toasted walnuts, chopped
	¼ cup fresh mint leaves
1 teaspoon canola oil	

1. Place the raisins in a small bowl. Pour 1 cup hot water over the raisins and let stand for 10 minutes, or until plumped. Drain well.

2. In a large bowl, whisk together the vinegar, pickled ginger, ginger juice, oil, and salt. Add the carrots, walnuts, mint, and raisins. Toss to mix well.

Nutrition per serving: 173 calories, 3 g protein, 19 g carbohydrates, 11 g total fat, 1 g saturated fat, 3 g fiber, 114 mg sodium

Make It a FLAT BELLY DIET MEAL

Serve with a grilled turkey burger (150), cut into slices, and ½ cup grilled baby red potatoes (75).
TOTAL MEAL: 398 calories

Heirloom Tomato Salad with Lemon Aioli

▥ PREP TIME: 15 MINUTES ▥ TOTAL TIME: 15 MINUTES ▥ MAKES 4 SERVINGS
▥ MUFA: CANOLA OIL MAYONNAISE

Enjoy this delicious combination in the summer when heirloom tomatoes are at their peak.

¼ cup canola oil mayonnaise
1 tablespoon lemon juice
½ teaspoon grated lemon peel
½ teaspoon gluten-free Dijon mustard
1 clove garlic, minced

2 medium heirloom tomatoes, thinly sliced
½ small red onion, cut into thin slivers
¼ cup basil leaves
2 teaspoons capers, rinsed and drained

1. In a small bowl, whisk together the mayonnaise, lemon juice, lemon peel, mustard, and garlic.

2. Arrange the tomato slices on 4 salad plates. Use the back of a spoon to spread equal portions of the aioli on the tomatoes. Scatter the onion over the aioli. Sprinkle with the basil and capers.

Nutrition per serving: 58 calories, 4 g fat, 0.5 g saturated fat, 1 g protein, 5 g carbohydrates, 1 g fiber, 176 mg sodium

Make It a FLAT BELLY DIET MEAL
Serve with Pizza Puttanesca (page 163), omitting the olives (206), and topped with 2 ounces gluten-free lean Italian turkey sausage (70) and an additional ¼ cup shredded, reduced-fat mozzarella cheese (70). TOTAL MEAL: 404 calories

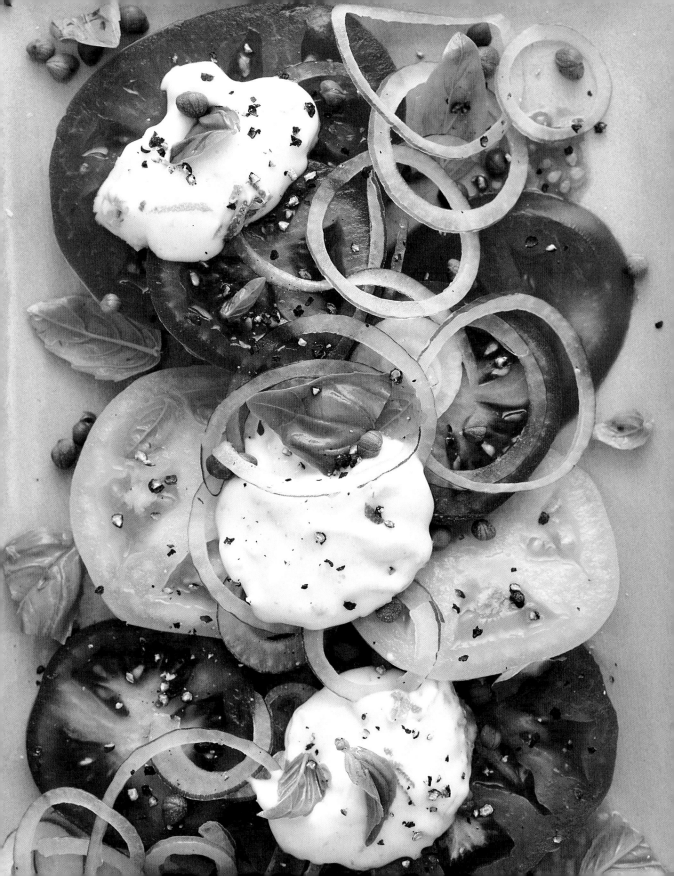

Broccoli-Pecan Salad

PREP TIME: 10 MINUTES ▓ TOTAL TIME: 15 MINUTES ▓ MAKES 4 SERVINGS ▓ MUFA: PECANS

Here's a popular potluck side salad, rendered perfect for a gluten-free Flat Belly Diet meal. For best results, make sure the florets are cut into small, uniform pieces.

2 cups small broccoli florets	1 cup cherry tomatoes, halved
3 tablespoons canola oil mayonnaise	1/2 cup unsalted toasted pecans
1 tablespoon white wine vinegar	1 shallot, finely chopped
Pinch of salt	

1. Bring a medium pot of water to a boil over high heat. Add the broccoli, reduce the heat to medium, cover, and simmer for 3 minutes, or until tender-crisp. Drain, rinse under cold running water, and drain again.

2. In a large bowl, combine the mayonnaise, vinegar, and salt. Add the broccoli, tomatoes, pecans, and shallot and toss to coat well.

Nutrition per serving: 203 calories, 3 g protein, 8 g carbohydrates, 19 g total fat, 1.5 g saturated fat, 3 g fiber, 152 mg sodium

Make It a FLAT BELLY DIET MEAL
Serve with Smoky Pork and Sweet Potato Skillet (page 210), omitting the avocado sauce (209).
TOTAL MEAL: 412 calories

Fennel and Grapefruit Salad

■ PREP TIME: 25 MINUTES ■ TOTAL TIME: 25 MINUTES ■ MAKES 4 SERVINGS
■ MUFA: OLIVES, WALNUT OIL

Top this refreshing salad with pan-seared or grilled shrimp or scallops.

2 ruby red grapefruits	1 large fennel bulb, thinly sliced
2 tablespoons walnut oil	20 oil-cured black olives, pitted and chopped
1 tablespoon gluten-free rice vinegar	¼ cup chopped fresh mint
¼ teaspoon coarsely ground black pepper	

1. With a small knife, cut away the peel and white pith from each grapefruit. Working over a small bowl, cut the flesh into segments, cutting them out of their membranes into the bowl. Squeeze the juice from the membranes. With a slotted spoon, transfer the grapefruit segments to a large bowl, leaving the juice behind. Add the oil, vinegar, and pepper to the small bowl and whisk with the juice.

2. Add the fennel, olives, and mint to the grapefruit sections. Drizzle with the juice mixture, tossing gently to coat well.

Nutrition per serving: 145 calories, 2 g protein, 19 g carbohydrates, 9 g total fat, 0.5 g saturated fat, 3 g fiber, 178 mg sodium

Make It a FLAT BELLY DIET MEAL

Serve with ½ cup cooked quinoa (111) and 3 ounces roasted chicken breast (140).
TOTAL MEAL: 396 calories

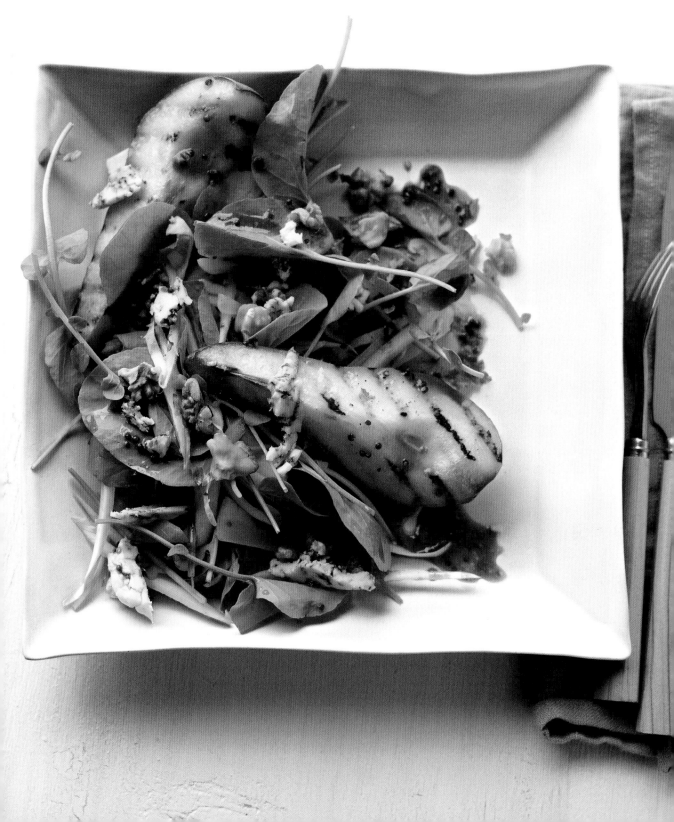

Grilled Pear Salad with Walnuts and Pomegranate Vinaigrette

▓ PREP TIME: 20 MINUTES ▓ TOTAL TIME: 30 MINUTES ▓ MAKES 4 SERVINGS ▓ MUFA: WALNUTS

For the best flavor, be sure to use firm ripe pears. If the pears are not quite ripe, place them in a bowl with apples or bananas, and store at room temperature for a day or two. The ethylene given off by the fruit will help to speed up the ripening process.

2 Bosc or Anjou pears, quartered and cored

2 tablespoons unsweetened pomegranate juice

1 tablespoon white wine vinegar

1 teaspoon olive oil

1 teaspoon honey

1 teaspoon gluten-free stone-ground mustard

¼ teaspoon salt

1 bunch watercress, trimmed

1 head Belgian endive, cored and thinly sliced

½ cup walnuts, toasted and chopped

4 tablespoons gluten-free crumbled blue or gorgonzola cheese

1. Coat a grill rack or nonstick grill pan with cooking spray and preheat to medium.

2. Lightly coat the pears with cooking spray. Place, cut side down, on the grill rack and grill until tender and well-marked, about 3 minutes on each side. Transfer the pears to a plate.

3. In a large bowl, whisk together the pomegranate juice, vinegar, oil, honey, mustard, and salt until blended. Add the watercress and endive and toss to coat evenly.

4. Divide the watercress mixture evenly among 4 plates. Top each with 2 pear wedges, 2 tablespoons of the walnuts, and 1 tablespoon of the cheese.

Nutrition per serving: 206 calories, 5 g protein, 24 g carbohydrates, 12 g total fat, 2.5 g saturated fat, 5 g fiber, 297 mg sodium

Make It a FLAT BELLY DIET MEAL Serve with Turkey Cutlets with Bacon and Avocado (page 192), omitting the avocado sauce (151), and 4 gluten-free multiseed crackers (35).
TOTAL MEAL: 392 calories

Curried Chicken Waldorf Salad

▓ PREP TIME: 15 MINUTES ▓ TOTAL TIME: 15 MINUTES ▓ MAKES 4 SERVINGS ▓ MUFA: WALNUTS

This salad offers the perfect opportunity to transform leftovers like chicken and brown rice into a completely new dish.

½ cup 0% plain Greek yogurt

2 tablespoons light mayonnaise

1 tablespoon curry powder

2 cups cooked cubed chicken breast

2 cups cooked brown rice

2 ribs celery, chopped

1 Granny Smith apple, chopped

½ cup toasted walnuts, coarsely chopped

¼ cup dried cranberries

2 tablespoons chopped fresh parsley

In a large bowl, whisk together the yogurt, mayonnaise, and curry powder until smooth. Add the chicken, rice, celery, apple, walnuts, cranberries, and parsley. Toss to mix well. Serve chilled or at room temperature.

Nutrition per serving: 395 calories, 29 g protein, 38 g carbohydrates, 14 g total fat, 2 g saturated fat, 5 g fiber, 158 mg sodium

Make It a FLAT BELLY DIET MEAL } A single serving of this recipe counts as a Flat Belly Diet Meal without any add-ons!

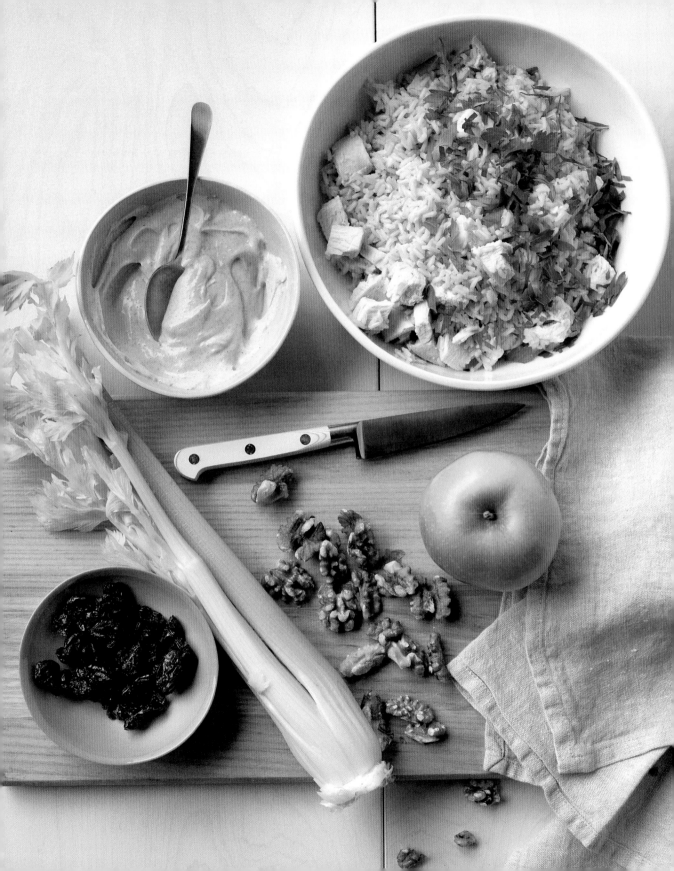

Pesto Chicken Caesar Salad

■ PREP TIME: 15 MINUTES ■ TOTAL TIME: 20 MINUTES ■ MAKES 4 SERVINGS ■ MUFA: OLIVE OIL

It's time to rethink the traditional Caesar salad. A crispy brown rice tortilla replaces standard croutons for a lighter crunch.

1 brown rice tortilla (8″ diameter)

¼ cup olive oil

2 teaspoons grated Romano cheese

2 hard-cooked eggs, peeled (discard 1 yolk)

2 tablespoons lemon juice

1½ tablespoons Pesto (page 84) or store-bought gluten-free pesto

½ teaspoon anchovy paste

6 cups torn romaine lettuce

2 cups cooked cubed chicken breast

Ground black pepper

1. Preheat the broiler. Brush the tortilla with a small amount of the oil. Sprinkle with the cheese. Place on a sheet of foil. Broil 6″ from the heat source for about 1 minute, or until golden and crisp. Remove from the oven and cut into small squares. Set aside.

2. Coarsely chop the egg whites and set aside.

3. In a large bowl, smash the egg yolk with a fork against the side of the bowl. Whisk in the lemon juice, pesto, anchovy paste, and the remaining oil until smooth. Add the romaine, chicken, and the reserved egg whites. Toss to coat well. Season generously with the pepper.

4. Scatter the tortilla pieces over the salad before serving.

Nutrition per serving: 339 calories, 27 g protein, 10 g carbohydrates, 21 g total fat, 4 g saturated fat, 2 g fiber, 287 mg sodium

Make It a
FLAT
BELLY
DIET
MEAL

Serve with 1 cup cantaloupe balls (60).
TOTAL MEAL: 399 calories

Tarragon Egg Salad Platter

▓ PREP TIME: 20 MINUTES ▓ TOTAL TIME: 20 MINUTES ▓ MAKES 4 SERVINGS
▓ MUFA: CANOLA OIL MAYONNAISE

Try this delicious platter in lieu of a conventional egg salad sandwich. Make sure to use canola mayonnaise, which draws its MUFA status from its main ingredient, canola oil.

6 hard-cooked eggs, peeled (discard 3 yolks)	½ teaspoon ground black pepper
3 ribs celery, chopped	Pinch of salt
3 scallions, thinly sliced	Leaf lettuce
¼ cup canola oil mayonnaise	2 large tomatoes, cut into wedges
1 tablespoon chopped fresh tarragon	8 gluten-free caraway crackers
½ teaspoon gluten-free coarse mustard	

1. Coarsely chop the eggs. Place them in a medium bowl and add the celery, scallions, mayonnaise, tarragon, mustard, pepper, and salt. Toss to mix well.

2. Arrange the lettuce leaves on a platter. Mound the salad on top and surround with the tomato wedges. Serve with the crackers.

Nutrition per serving: 223 calories, 9 g protein, 11 g carbohydrates, 16 g total fat, 2 g saturated fat, 3 g fiber, 338 mg sodium

Make It a
FLAT
BELLY
DIET
MEAL
} Serve with Cashew Brownies (page 268), omitting the cashews (192).
TOTAL MEAL: 415 calories

Minted Watermelon Salad with Avocado

■ PREP TIME: 15 MINUTES ■ TOTAL TIME: 15 MINUTES ■ MAKES 4 SERVINGS ■ MUFA: AVOCADO

This delicious combination tastes best the day it's made. Serve it chilled for the best flavor.

2 tablespoons lime juice

1 tablespoon olive oil

¼ teaspoon salt

1 small seedless watermelon (about 4 pounds), cut into 1½" chunks

1 Hass avocado, peeled, pitted, and chopped

½ small red onion, thinly sliced

3 tablespoons chopped fresh mint

In a large bowl, whisk together the lime juice, oil, and salt. Add the watermelon, avocado, onion, and mint, and toss gently to mix.

Nutrition per serving: 204 calories, 3 g protein, 32 g carbohydrates, 9 g total fat, 1 g saturated fat, 4 g fiber, 154 mg sodium

Make It a
FLAT
BELLY
DIET
MEAL

Serve with Curried Cashew Chicken (page 184), omitting the cashews (196).

TOTAL MEAL: 400 calories

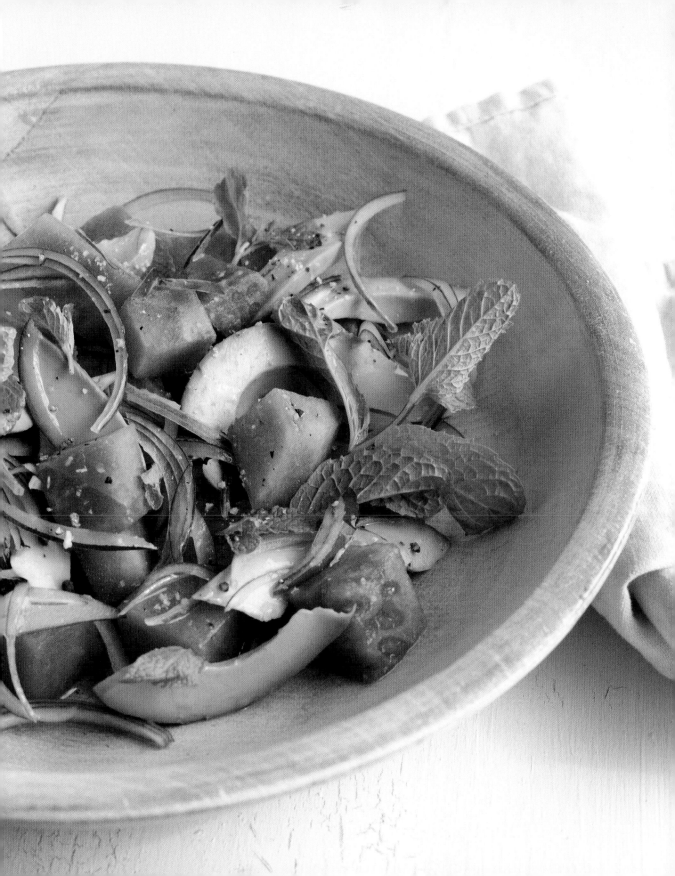

Crunchy Bell Pepper and Cucumber Slaw

■ PREP TIME: 20 MINUTES ■ TOTAL TIME: 20 MINUTES ■ MAKES 4 SERVINGS ■ MUFA: PEANUTS

Make a double batch of the peanut dressing and use it as a basting sauce for grilled chicken skewers. Mirin adds a bit of sweetness to the dressing, but you can use 1 teaspoon of honey instead.

2 tablespoons creamy natural peanut butter

2 tablespoons gluten-free rice vinegar

1 tablespoon gluten-free mirin

1 tablespoon grated peeled fresh ginger

1 tablespoon gluten-free reduced-sodium soy sauce

1 red bell pepper, cut into thin strips

½ small hothouse (seedless) cucumber, cut into thin strips

1 cup bean sprouts

4 scallions, thinly sliced

½ cup unsalted dry-roasted peanuts, chopped

In a large bowl, whisk together the peanut butter, vinegar, mirin, ginger, and soy sauce until smooth. Add the bell pepper, cucumber, bean sprouts, scallions, and peanuts and toss until well coated.

Nutrition per serving: 200 calories, 8 g protein, 14 g carbohydrates, 13 g total fat, 2 g saturated fat, 4 g fiber, 216 mg sodium

Make It a
FLAT
BELLY
DIET
MEAL

Serve with 3 ounces roasted center-cut pork loin (217).
TOTAL MEAL: 417 calories

Asian Chopped Salad
with Spicy Peanut Dressing

■ PREP TIME: 15 MINUTES ■ TOTAL TIME: 20 MINUTES ■ MAKES 4 SERVINGS
■ MUFA: PEANUTS, PEANUT BUTTER

**Everything for this salad can be prepared ahead of time. Make the dressing
and store in an airtight container for up to 3 days. Prepare the vegetables
(except the bean sprouts) and keep them in a resealable food storage bag in
the refrigerator up to 2 days. Top with the bean sprouts and peanuts just
before serving.**

1 bag (10 ounces) frozen shelled
 edamame

3 tablespoons gluten-free
 rice vinegar

2 tablespoons creamy natural
 peanut butter

2 tablespoons gluten-free
 reduced-sodium soy sauce

2 tablespoons warm water

¼ teaspoon red-pepper flakes

2 cups shredded Napa or
 Savoy cabbage

1 red bell pepper, chopped

1 cup loosely packed cilantro leaves

1 cup bean sprouts

6 tablespoons unsalted dry-roasted
 peanuts, coarsely chopped

1. Bring a large pot of water to a boil over high heat. Add the edamame and cook for
5 minutes, or until bright green. Drain, run under cold running water, and drain again.

2. Meanwhile, in a large bowl, whisk together the vinegar, peanut butter, soy sauce,
water, and red-pepper flakes until smooth. Add the edamame, cabbage, bell pepper,
and cilantro. Toss to coat well. Top with the bean sprouts and sprinkle with the peanuts.

Nutrition per serving: 242 calories, 15 g protein, 17 g carbohydrates, 14 g total fat, 1.5 g saturated fat,
7 g fiber, 359 mg sodium

Make It a
FLAT
BELLY
DIET
MEAL

Serve with 4 ounces steamed shrimp (112) and 1 clementine (35).
TOTAL MEAL: 389 calories

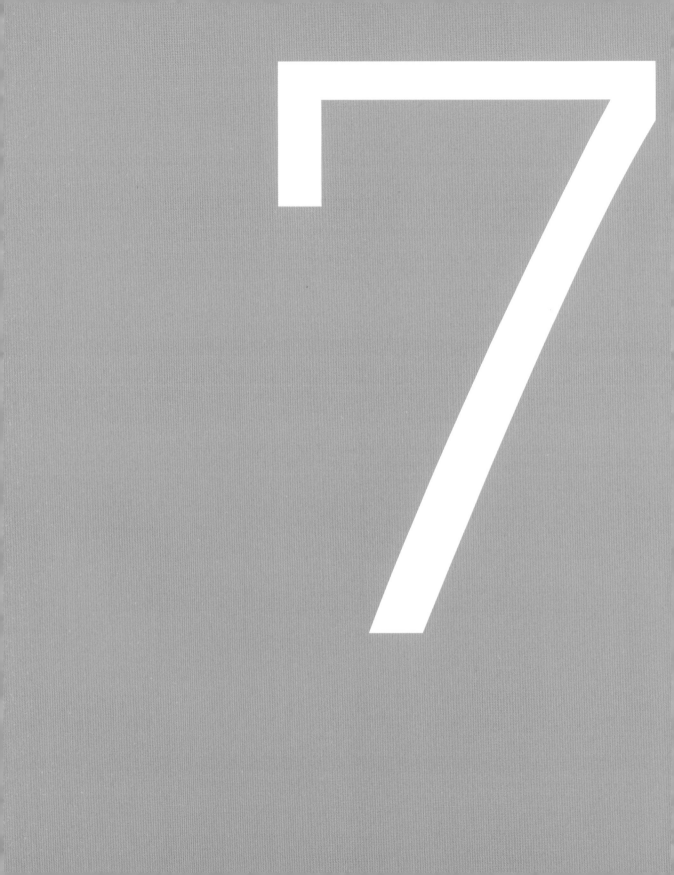

VEGETARIAN

Garlicky Grilled Tofu Cutlets with Vegetables

▓ PREP TIME: 10 MINUTES ▓ TOTAL TIME: 25 MINUTES ▓ MAKES 4 SERVINGS ▓ MUFA: WALNUT OIL

Too often tofu gets a bad rap for bland flavor, but so would chicken breast if it weren't seasoned. This dish should set the record straight on tofu's ability to taste great.

1 large yellow or red bell pepper, finely chopped

4 scallions, white and green parts, finely chopped

2 small ribs celery, finely chopped

2 cloves garlic, minced

4 tablespoons walnut oil, divided

1 container (14 ounces) extra-firm tofu, drained and cut into 4 pieces

1 teaspoon salt-free garlic and herb seasoning blend, divided

2 teaspoons red wine vinegar

¼ teaspoon salt

1 package (5 ounces) shredded red cabbage (about 2 cups)

1. Preheat the grill to medium.

2. Toss the bell pepper, scallions, celery, garlic, and 1 tablespoon of the oil in a 13″ x 9″ shallow disposable aluminum baking pan.

3. Push the vegetables to the edges of the pan and set the tofu slices in the center. Sprinkle with ½ teaspoon of the seasoning blend and 1½ teaspoons of the oil. Flip and sprinkle with the remaining ½ teaspoon seasoning blend and 1½ teaspoons of the oil.

4. Place the pan over direct heat and grill, turning the tofu once and stirring the vegetables occasionally, for 15 minutes, or until hot and sizzling.

5. Meanwhile, in a medium bowl, whisk together the vinegar, salt, and the remaining 2 tablespoons oil. Add the cabbage and toss to coat. Serve the cabbage topped with the tofu and vegetables.

Nutrition per serving: 249 calories, 11 g protein, 10 g carbohydrates, 19 g total fat, 3 g saturated fat, 3 g fiber, 170 mg sodium

Make It a FLAT BELLY DIET MEAL

Serve with ¾ cup cooked brown rice (145).
TOTAL MEAL: 394 calories

PERFECT TOFU EVERY TIME

If tofu was not a regular staple of your diet before, you may feel intimidated by those squishy white cubes of lean protein. But never fear: Just as with meat and poultry, there are special tricks to preparing outstanding tofu. Keep these three steps in mind:

O **Squeeze:** Extra-firm tofu typically comes packed in water, so you'll want to press excess moisture from the spongelike tofu before cooking—kind of like when you're opening a can of water-packed tuna. Since tofu isn't sold in a can, try this instead: Lay a kitchen towel or paper towels on your counter, place the tofu on top, and slice into however many pieces you need. Then use either your hand, covered in another towel, or a heavy object to push as much excess moisture out as possible. If you have time to prepare ahead, you can leave the heavy object sitting atop the tofu for 30 minutes or longer for maximum drainage.

O **Season or marinate:** To infuse your tofu with flavor, choose a non-oil-based marinade or simply sprinkle with your favorite seasoning before cooking. The more time the tofu has to soak up the ingredients, the better.

O **Grill:** Tofu is just processed soy, so unlike meat, it doesn't need to be cooked to a certain internal temperature. Just throw it on the grill (grease the grill with a bit of canola oil first!), and let your tofu cook until it gets crispy, with some lovely grill marks on the side.

Tofu, Asparagus, and Cashew Stir-Fry

■ PREP TIME: 15 MINUTES ■ TOTAL TIME: 25 MINUTES ■ MAKES 4 SERVINGS ■ MUFA: CASHEWS

Add ½ pound shiitake mushrooms to the stir-fry, if you like. Be sure to remove and discard their tough stems before using.

1½ cups gluten-free vegetable broth
1 tablespoon gluten-free rice vinegar
1 tablespoon gluten-free reduced-sodium soy sauce
2 teaspoons cornstarch
1 teaspoon toasted sesame oil
2 teaspoons peanut oil
4 scallions, cut into 3" pieces
1 tablespoon grated fresh ginger

2 cloves garlic, minced
¼ teaspoon red-pepper flakes
1 pound asparagus, cut into 2" pieces
1 package (14 ounces) firm tofu, cut into 1" pieces
½ cup roasted cashews, coarsely chopped

1. In a small bowl, whisk together the broth, vinegar, soy sauce, cornstarch, and sesame oil until smooth. Set aside.

2. In a large nonstick skillet over medium-high heat, warm the peanut oil. Add the scallions, ginger, garlic, and red-pepper flakes and cook, stirring, for 1 minute, or until fragrant. Add the asparagus and cook, stirring, for 3 minutes, or until tender-crisp.

3. Add the tofu, cashews, and broth mixture to the skillet. Cook, stirring, for 2 minutes, or until the sauce begins to bubble and thicken. Serve at once.

Nutrition per serving: 261 calories, 15 g protein, 17 g carbohydrates, 17 g total fat, 3 g saturated fat, 4 g fiber, 468 mg sodium

Make It a
FLAT
BELLY
DIET
MEAL

Serve with 1 medium baked sweet potato without skin (103) and 1 teaspoon trans-free margarine (27).
TOTAL MEAL: 391 calories

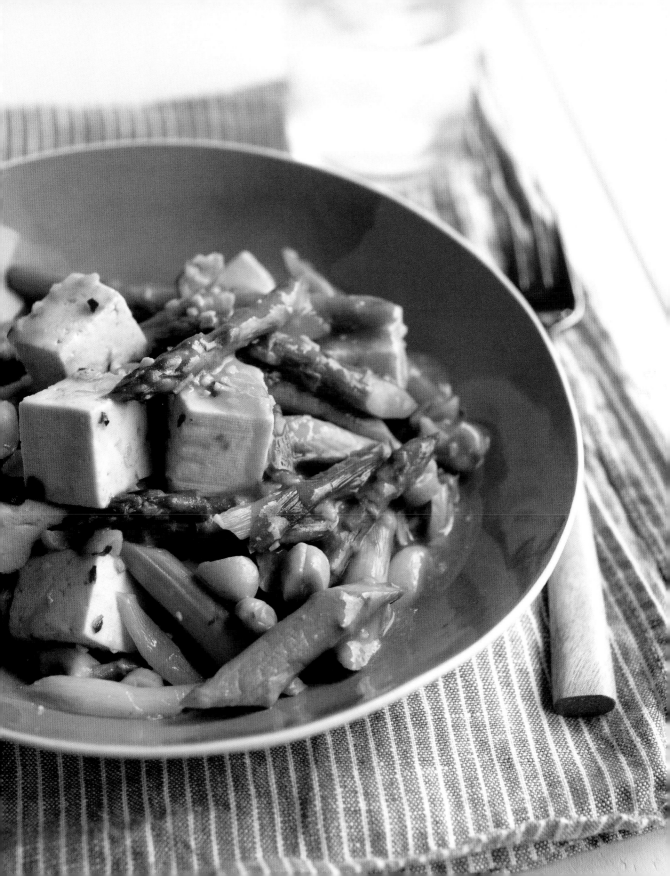

Eggplant Rolls with Roasted Red Peppers and Pesto

PREP TIME: 20 MINUTES ▥ **TOTAL TIME: 30 MINUTES** ▥ **MAKES 4 SERVINGS**
▥ **MUFA: PESTO, OLIVE OIL**

You will never miss breaded eggplant again with the bright fresh flavors in this dish. Serve with a tomato and cucumber salad.

1 eggplant (about 1 pound), cut lengthwise into 8 slices

2 tablespoons Pesto (page 84) or store-bought gluten-free pesto

½ cup roasted red pepper strips (from a jar), drained and patted dry

½ cup crumbled reduced-fat feta cheese

2 tablespoons olive oil

1 tablespoon lemon juice

1 tablespoon chopped fresh basil

¼ teaspoon salt

1. Heat a nonstick grill pan coated with cooking spray over medium-high heat. Lightly coat both sides of the eggplant slices with cooking spray. Cook the eggplant, in batches if necessary, about 4 minutes on each side, or until well-marked and tender. Transfer the eggplant to a work surface to cool slightly.

2. Brush each eggplant slice with ¾ teaspoon of the pesto. Top each evenly with the bell pepper strips and feta. Roll up and place, seam side down, on a platter.

3. In a small bowl, whisk together the oil, lemon juice, basil, and salt. Drizzle over the rolls. Serve at once or cover and refrigerate up to 2 hours.

Nutrition per serving: 172 calories, 6 g protein, 10 g carbohydrates, 13 g total fat, 3.5 g saturated fat, 4 g fiber, 592 mg sodium

Make It a FLAT BELLY DIET MEAL

Serve with 1 cup cooked quinoa (222).
TOTAL MEAL: 394 calories

Pizza Puttanesca

■ PREP TIME: 10 MINUTES ■ TOTAL TIME: 25 MINUTES ■ MAKES 6 SERVINGS (2 SLICES EACH)
■ MUFA: OLIVES

These savory pies are excellent when you need to get dinner on the table quickly! For some extra authentic Italian flavor, sprinkle garlic powder or red-pepper flakes onto the baked pizzas before serving.

2 gluten-free thin pizza crusts (8"–9" diameter)

½ cup gluten-free marinara sauce

40 kalamata olives, pitted and chopped

2 tablespoons olive oil

2 teaspoons capers, rinsed and drained

½ cup shredded reduced-fat mozzarella cheese

¼ cup chopped fresh basil

1. Preheat the oven according to the pizza crust package directions. Coat a large baking sheet with cooking spray. Prebake the crusts, if directed.

2. Spread the sauce evenly over the crusts. Top each with half of the olives, half of the oil, and half of the capers. Sprinkle with the cheese.

3. Bake for 10 to 12 minutes, or until the crust is crisp and the cheese is melted. Sprinkle with the basil and cut each pizza into 6 wedges.

Nutrition per serving: 277 calories, 6 g protein, 26 g carbohydrates, 16 g total fat, 2 g saturated fat, 1 g fiber, 811 mg sodium

Make It a
FLAT
BELLY
DIET
MEAL

Serve with 2 cups salad greens with 2 tablespoons balsamic vinaigrette (98).
TOTAL MEAL: 375 calories

Mushroom, Onion, and Avocado Quesadillas

■ PREP TIME: 10 MINUTES ■ TOTAL TIME: 35 MINUTES ■ MAKES 4 SERVINGS ■ MUFA: AVOCADO

If your family is addicted to taco night, switch things up and try a quesadilla night instead. These meaty-tasting mushrooms are so satisfying you're likely to have a new tradition on your hands.

1 tablespoon olive oil
¼ pound cremini mushrooms, sliced
¼ pound shiitake mushrooms, tough stems removed, caps sliced
1 onion, chopped
4 cloves garlic, minced
¼ teaspoon salt

1 Hass avocado, peeled, pitted, and chopped
2 tablespoons chopped fresh cilantro
4 gluten-free brown rice tortillas (8″ diameter)
1 cup shredded reduced-fat sharp Cheddar cheese

1. In a large nonstick skillet over medium-high heat, warm the oil. Add the mushrooms, onion, garlic, and salt and cook, stirring occasionally, for 8 minutes, or until browned.

2. In a small bowl, coarsely mash the avocado and stir in the cilantro. Arrange the tortillas in a single layer on a work surface. Spread the bottom half of each tortilla with one-fourth of the avocado mixture. Top each with 2 tablespoons of the cheese and one-fourth of the mushroom mixture. Sprinkle each with 2 tablespoons of the remaining cheese. Fold the top half of each tortilla over the filling.

3. Wipe out the skillet, coat it with cooking spray, and place over medium-high heat. Cook 2 quesadillas for 3 to 4 minutes per side, or until the filling is hot and the outside is lightly browned. Repeat with the remaining quesadillas. Transfer to a cutting board and cut each in half before serving.

Nutrition per serving: 296 calories, 11 g protein, 29 g carbohydrates, 17 g total fat, 5 g saturated fat, 5 g fiber, 504 mg sodium

Make It a
FLAT
BELLY
DIET
MEAL

Serve with 1 cup sliced mango (107).
TOTAL MEAL: 403 calories

White Bean and Spinach Ragu with Polenta

■ PREP TIME: 15 MINUTES ■ TOTAL TIME: 35 MINUTES ■ MAKES 4 SERVINGS
■ MUFA: BLACK OLIVE TAPENADE

Cheesy, soft polenta makes the perfect base for this hearty white bean stew. Use leftover Pan-Fried Cheesy Polenta (page 79) to save time and ingredients!

2 tablespoons olive oil

1 onion, finely chopped

1 teaspoon dried oregano

3 cloves garlic, minced

1 can (15 ounces) no-salt-added cannellini beans, rinsed and drained

1 can (14.5 ounces) no-salt-added diced tomatoes

1 bag (5 ounces) baby spinach

½ cup Black Olive Tapenade (page 80) or store-bought gluten-free tapenade

2 cups 1% milk

1 cup water

¼ teaspoon salt

½ cup gluten-free instant polenta

¼ cup grated Parmesan cheese

1. In a large nonstick skillet over medium-high heat, warm the oil. Add the onion and oregano and cook, stirring occasionally, for 2 to 3 minutes, or until the onion begins to soften. Stir in the garlic and cook for 30 seconds. Add the beans and cook for 3 minutes. Stir in the tomatoes and cook for 3 to 4 minutes, or until starting to thicken. Add the spinach and cook, stirring, for 2 to 3 minutes, or until the spinach just begins to wilt. Stir in the tapenade. Remove from the heat and keep warm.

2. In a medium saucepan, bring the milk, water, and salt to a boil over high heat. Whisking constantly, gradually add the instant polenta in a slow steady stream until the mixture is smooth and free from any lumps. Reduce the heat to medium and cook, stirring constantly with a wooden spoon, for 5 minutes, or until the mixture is thick. Remove from the heat and stir in the cheese.

3. Serve the ragu on top of the polenta.

Nutrition per serving: 389 calories, 14 g protein, 54 g carbohydrates, 15 g total fat, 3 g saturated fat, 8 g fiber, 583 mg sodium

Make It a FLAT BELLY DIET MEAL A single serving of this recipe counts as a Flat Belly Diet Meal without any add-ons!

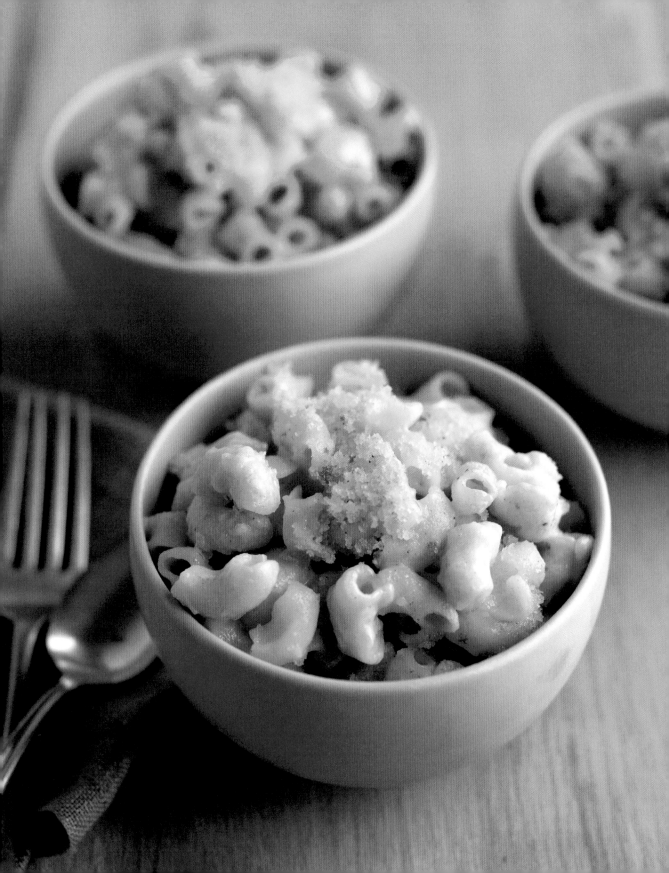

Old-Fashioned Mac 'n' Cheese

■ PREP TIME: 10 MINUTES ■ TOTAL TIME: 40 MINUTES ■ MAKES 4 SERVINGS ■ MUFA: OLIVE OIL

You probably won't have any trouble enticing your family to eat this creamy macaroni and cheese casserole. You can even keep the MUFA a secret if you want.

4 ounces gluten-free quinoa elbow pasta

3 tablespoons gluten-free bread crumbs

4 tablespoons olive oil, divided

2 tablespoons gluten-free all-purpose flour

½ teaspoon paprika

½ teaspoon salt

2 cups fat-free milk

½ cup shredded reduced-fat Cheddar cheese

1. Preheat the oven to 350°F. Coat an 8" x 8" baking dish with cooking spray.

2. Bring a medium pot of water to a boil. Add the pasta and cook according to package directions. Drain, rinse with cold water, and drain again. Set aside.

3. In a small bowl, combine the bread crumbs and 2 teaspoons of the oil with a fork until evenly coated.

4. In a large saucepan over medium-high heat, warm the remaining oil. Whisk in the flour, paprika, and salt until smooth. Gradually whisk in the milk, whisking constantly. Cook, whisking, for 5 minutes, or until thickened. Remove from the heat. Stir in the cheese until melted. Stir in the reserved pasta. Pour into the prepared baking dish. Top evenly with the crumb mixture.

5. Bake for 15 minutes, or until the edges are bubbly and the topping is browned. Let stand for 10 minutes before serving.

Nutrition per serving: 343 calories, 10 g protein, 37 g carbohydrates, 18 g total fat, 3.5 g saturated fat, 3 g fiber, 484 mg sodium

Make It a
FLAT
BELLY
DIET
MEAL
} Serve with 1 cup of steamed broccoli (55).
TOTAL MEAL: 398 calories

Fettuccine with Broccoli Pesto

■ PREP TIME: 10 MINUTES ■ TOTAL TIME: 25 MINUTES ■ MAKES 4 SERVINGS
■ MUFA: PINE NUTS, OLIVE OIL

If you like, add 1 cup frozen peas to the pasta during the last 2 minutes of cooking time. Drain the pasta and peas together before tossing with the pesto.

8 ounces brown rice fettuccine or linguine pasta	2 tablespoons grated Parmesan cheese
2 cups small broccoli florets	2 tablespoons olive oil
1 cup fresh basil leaves	2 cloves garlic, halved
¼ cup pine nuts	¼ teaspoon salt

1. Cook the pasta according to package directions. Drain, rinse under warm running water, and drain again. Place the pasta in a large bowl.

2. Meanwhile, place a steamer basket in a large saucepan with 2" of water. Bring to a boil, add the broccoli, and steam for 3 to 4 minutes, or until tender-crisp. Drain under cold running water and drain again.

3. In a food processor, place the broccoli, basil, pine nuts, cheese, oil, garlic, and salt. Pulse until smooth. Add the pesto to the pasta in the bowl and toss to coat well.

Nutrition per serving: 352 calories, 8 g protein, 46 g carbohydrates, 14 g total fat, 2 g saturated fat, 3 g fiber, 194 mg sodium

Make It a FLAT BELLY DIET MEAL

Serve with 1 cup steamed asparagus (40).
TOTAL MEAL: 392 calories

Double-Stuffed Mushrooms with Lentils and Walnuts

■ PREP TIME: 10 MINUTES ■ TOTAL TIME: 50 MINUTES ■ MAKES 4 SERVINGS ■ MUFA: WALNUTS

You can prepare the filling up to 2 days ahead of time, then fill and bake the mushrooms right before serving.

2½ cups water

⅓ cup brown lentils

1 tablespoon olive oil

½ pound shiitake mushrooms, tough stems removed, caps sliced

1 onion, chopped

2 cloves garlic, chopped

½ cup toasted chopped walnuts

1 teaspoon chopped fresh rosemary

½ teaspoon salt

½ cup shredded Gouda cheese, divided

4 portobello mushroom caps, 4" diameter (about 3 ounces each)

1. In a medium saucepan, bring the water to a boil over high heat. Add the lentils and reduce to a simmer. Cover and cook for 20 minutes, or just until tender. Drain well and cool.

2. Meanwhile, in a medium nonstick skillet, heat the oil over medium-high heat. Add the shiitake mushrooms, onion, and garlic and cook, stirring occasionally, for 5 minutes, or until tender. Remove from the heat and let cool slightly.

3. Preheat the oven to 400°F. Coat a small rimmed baking sheet with cooking spray.

4. In a food processor, place the lentils, shiitake mushroom mixture, walnuts, rosemary, salt, and ¼ cup of the cheese. Pulse until coarsely chopped. Fill the mushroom caps with the mixture, mounding slightly. Top with the remaining ¼ cup cheese.

5. Place on the prepared baking sheet and bake for 20 minutes, or until the filling is heated through and the topping is lightly browned.

Nutrition per serving: 264 calories, 12 g protein, 19 g carbohydrates, 18 g total fat, 4 g saturated fat, 7 g fiber, 423 mg sodium

Make It a FLAT BELLY DIET MEAL } Serve with 1 medium apple sliced into wedges (95) and drizzled with 1 teaspoon honey (20).
TOTAL MEAL: 379 calories

SEAFOOD

Halibut with Chopped Olive and Potato Salad

■ PREP TIME: 10 MINUTES ■ TOTAL TIME: 20 MINUTES ■ MAKES 4 SERVINGS ■ MUFA: OLIVES

Halibut is an excellent source of magnesium, a mineral that helps regulate blood sugar levels and promotes normal blood pressure.

20 large black olives, pitted and chopped

20 kalamata olives, pitted and chopped

1 cup cooked cubed potatoes

¼ cup finely chopped roasted red peppers (from a jar), drained

2 tablespoons finely chopped red onion

1 tablespoon chopped fresh basil

2 teaspoons white wine vinegar

5 teaspoons olive oil, divided

4 halibut fillets (6 ounces each)

1. In a medium bowl, combine the olives, potatoes, peppers, onion, basil, vinegar, and 3 teaspoons of the oil.

2. In a large nonstick skillet over medium-high heat, warm the remaining 2 teaspoons oil. Cook the fillets for 4 to 5 minutes per side, or until the fish flakes easily with a fork.

3. Divide the fish among 4 plates and top evenly with the olive mixture.

Nutrition per serving: 350 calories, 37 g protein, 11 g carbohydrates, 18 g total fat, 2 g saturated fat, 2 g fiber, 631 mg sodium

Make It a FLAT BELLY DIET MEAL

Serve with 1 cup steamed green beans (44).

TOTAL MEAL: 394 calories

Tilapia with Sizzling Sesame Scallions

■ PREP TIME: 5 MINUTES ■ TOTAL TIME: 20 MINUTES ■ MAKES 4 SERVINGS ■ MUFA: SESAME SEEDS

Tilapia, a firm whitefish that is quite versatile in the kitchen, is usually farm raised, making it a very sustainable seafood choice.

2 tablespoons lemon juice

1 tablespoon honey

¼ teaspoon salt

4 tilapia fillets (6 ounces each)

8 scallions, white and green parts, halved lengthwise, then cut on the diagonal into 1" pieces

½ cup sesame seeds

1. Preheat the grill to medium. Coat an 11" x 7" shallow disposable aluminum baking pan with cooking spray. Whisk in the lemon juice, honey, and salt.

2. Dip the fillets, one piece at a time, into the mixture to coat both sides and set on one side of the pan. Stir the scallions and sesame seeds into the remaining honey mixture, then push to the opposite side. Arrange the fillets in the middle of the pan with most of the sesame mixture surrounding them.

3. Place the pan on the grill over direct heat and grill, stirring the sesame mixture occasionally, for 5 to 6 minutes per side, or until the fish flakes easily and the sesame seeds have toasted. If necessary, transfer the fillets to a platter and continue cooking the sesame mixture for 1 to 2 minutes, or until the sesame seeds are browned. Serve the tilapia topped with the sesame mixture.

Nutrition per serving: 281 calories, 37 g protein, 11 g carbohydrates, 11 g total fat, 2 g saturated fat, 4 g fiber, 245 mg sodium

Make It a FLAT BELLY DIET MEAL

Serve with ½ cup cooked brown rice (109).
TOTAL MEAL: 390 calories

Pecan-Crusted Cod

■ PREP TIME: 15 MINUTES ■ TOTAL TIME: 30 MINUTES ■ MAKES 4 SERVINGS ■ MUFA: PECANS

The apricot-mustard mixture not only adds flavor, but keeps the fish moist while baking.

2 tablespoons apricot fruit spread

1 tablespoon gluten-free Dijon mustard

1 egg white

1 teaspoon cornstarch

½ cup unsalted pecans, finely chopped

½ cup gluten-free plain bread crumbs

4 cod fillets (5 ounces each)

½ teaspoon salt

1. Preheat the oven to 425°F. Coat a rimmed baking sheet with cooking spray.

2. In a medium bowl, whisk together the fruit spread, mustard, egg white, and cornstarch. Combine the pecans and bread crumbs on a sheet of waxed paper. Sprinkle the fillets with the salt. Dip the fillets, one piece at a time, into the fruit spread mixture, then into the crumb mixture, pressing to adhere.

3. Place the fillets on the baking sheet and lightly coat with cooking spray. Bake for 15 minutes, or until the fish flakes.

Nutrition per serving: 307 calories, 29 g protein, 20 g carbohydrates, 13 g total fat, 1 g saturated fat, 2 g fiber, 538 mg sodium

Make It a FLAT BELLY DIET MEAL

Serve with ½ cup grilled baby red potatoes (75).
TOTAL MEAL: 382 calories

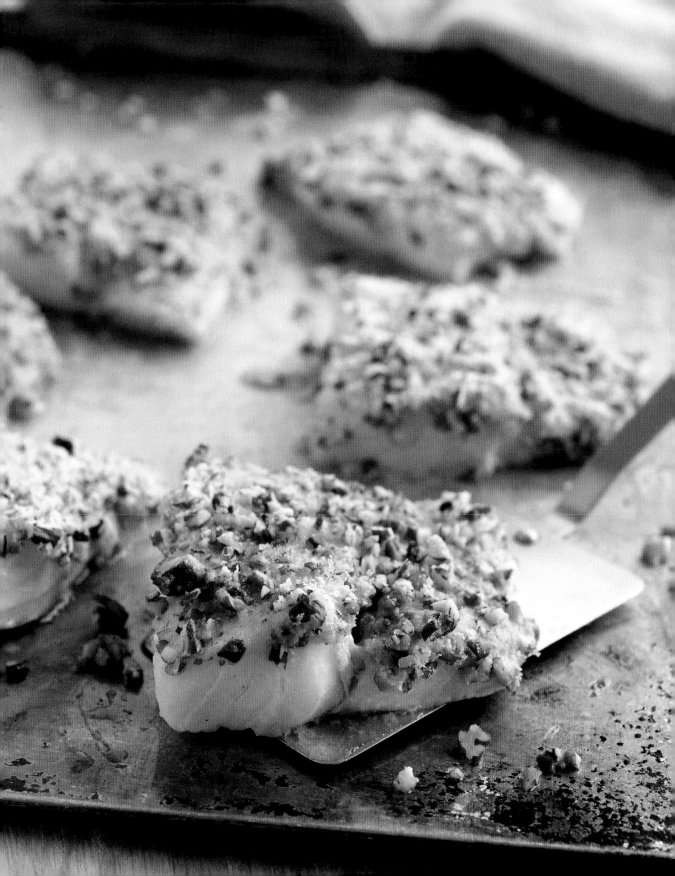

Sake-Steamed Sole with Baby Bok Choy

■ PREP TIME: 10 MINUTES ■ TOTAL TIME: 20 MINUTES ■ MAKES 4 SERVINGS
■ MUFA: SESAME SEEDS

Cod, tilapia, or any other firm whitefish may be used in place of the sole.

2 teaspoons toasted sesame oil

3 scallions, cut into 3" pieces

1 piece ginger (2"), thinly sliced

2 cloves garlic, thinly sliced

1/4 teaspoon red-pepper flakes

1 pound baby bok choy, halved lengthwise (about 6 heads)

1/4 cup gluten-free low-sodium chicken broth

1/4 cup gluten-free sake

1 tablespoon gluten-free soy sauce

1/2 cup toasted sesame seeds, divided

4 sole or flounder fillets (4 ounces each)

1. In a large skillet, heat the oil over medium-high heat. Add the scallions, ginger, garlic, and red-pepper flakes and cook, stirring, for 1 minute, or until fragrant. Add the bok choy (cut side down), broth, sake, soy sauce, and 1/4 cup of the sesame seeds. Cover and cook for 2 minutes, or until the bok choy begins to wilt.

2. Meanwhile, spread the remaining 1/4 cup sesame seeds on a sheet of waxed paper and press the fish firmly onto the seeds. Tuck in the ends of each fillet and place on top of the bok choy in the skillet. Cover and simmer for 5 minutes, or until the bok choy is tender-crisp and the fish flakes easily.

Nutrition per serving: 263 calories, 27 g protein, 10 g carbohydrates, 12 g total fat, 2 g saturated fat, 4 g fiber, 434 mg sodium

Make It a FLAT BELLY DIET MEAL

Serve with 1 cup of steamed broccoli (20) and 2/3 cup cooked brown rice (130).

TOTAL MEAL: 413 calories

Portuguese Shellfish Stew

■ PREP TIME: 15 MINUTES ■ TOTAL TIME: 45 MINUTES
■ MAKES 4 SERVINGS (2¾ CUPS EACH) ■ MUFA: OLIVE OIL

Any variety of seafood can be used here. Scallops, cod, and crabmeat work well. If you feel like indulging, add some lobster.

¼ cup olive oil, divided

1 pound mussels, scrubbed and debearded

1 dozen littleneck clams, scrubbed

½ pound large shrimp, peeled and deveined

1 can (28 ounces) no-salt-added Italian peeled tomatoes

¾ cup gluten-free low-sodium chicken broth

½ cup dry white wine

3 cloves garlic, thinly sliced

½ teaspoon salt

¼ teaspoon red-pepper flakes

½ cup chopped fresh basil

1. In a large skillet over medium-high heat, warm 1 tablespoon of the oil. Cook the mussels and clams, covered, for about 4 minutes for the mussels, and about 9 minutes for the clams, or until they begin to open. With tongs, transfer the mussels and clams to a large bowl as they open. Discard any that do not open. Cover the bowl loosely with foil.

2. Add the shrimp to the skillet and cook for 4 minutes, turning occasionally, or until the shrimp begin to turn opaque. Transfer to the bowl with the mussels and clams.

3. Add the remaining 3 tablespoons oil to the skillet along with the tomatoes, broth, wine, garlic, salt, and red-pepper flakes and bring to a boil. Cook, partially covered and stirring occasionally, for 15 minutes, or until the sauce thickens slightly and the flavors are blended.

4. Return the seafood to the skillet and heat through. Remove from the heat. Stir in the basil.

Nutrition per serving: 386 calories, 33 g protein, 16 g carbohydrates, 18 g total fat, 3 g saturated fat, 2 g fiber, 594 mg sodium

Make It a
FLAT
BELLY
DIET
MEAL
} A single serving of this recipe counts as a Flat Belly Diet Meal without any add-ons!

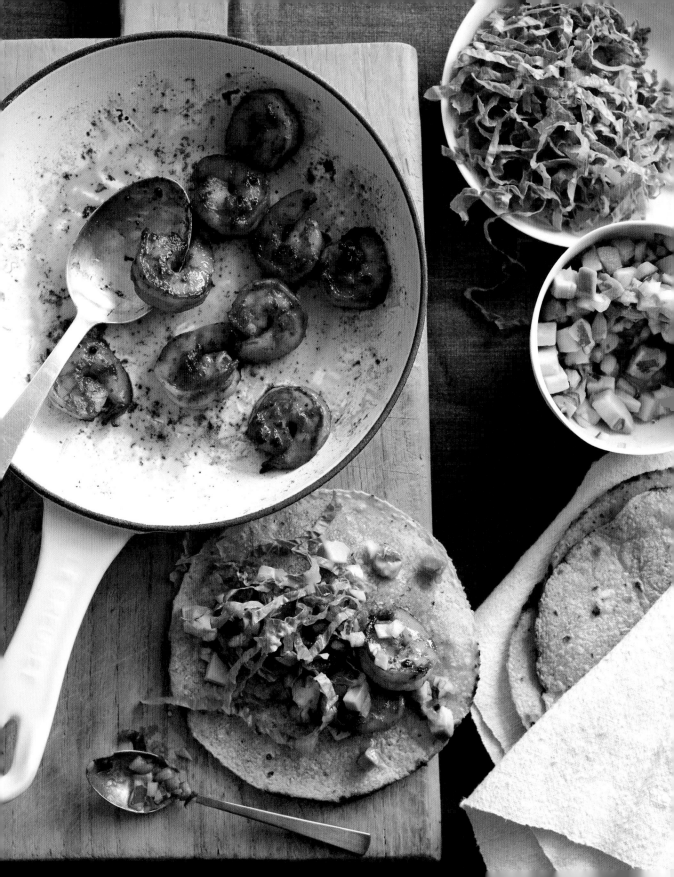

Fiery Shrimp Tacos

■ PREP TIME: 10 MINUTES ■ TOTAL TIME: 20 MINUTES ■ MAKES 4 SERVINGS ■ MUFA: AVOCADO

Not batter-dipped or deep-fried, as many fish tacos are, these leaner tacos are loaded with heart-healthy MUFAs from the avocado topping.

1 Hass avocado, peeled, pitted, and cubed

3 tablespoons finely chopped red onion

2 tablespoons chopped fresh cilantro

½ jalapeño chile pepper, finely chopped (wear plastic gloves when handling)

1 tablespoon lime juice

½ teaspoon salt, divided

1 pound peeled and deveined medium shrimp

1½ teaspoons chili powder

1 tablespoon olive oil

8 gluten-free corn tortillas (6" diameter)

1 cup shredded romaine lettuce

1. In a small bowl, combine the avocado, onion, cilantro, chile pepper, lime juice, and ¼ teaspoon of the salt until blended. Set aside.

2. In a medium bowl, toss the shrimp with the chili powder and the remaining ¼ teaspoon salt.

3. In a large nonstick skillet over medium-high heat, warm the oil. Cook the shrimp for 2½ to 3 minutes per side, or until opaque. Transfer to a plate and keep warm.

4. Wipe out the skillet. Heat the tortillas over medium-high heat for about 30 seconds per side, or according to package directions, until hot and lightly toasted. Top each tortilla evenly with the romaine, the reserved avocado mixture, and the shrimp. Serve hot.

Nutrition per serving: 317 calories, 26 g protein, 23 g carbohydrates, 14 g total fat, 2 g saturated fat, 6 g fiber, 474 mg sodium

Make It a
FLAT
BELLY
DIET
MEAL
} Serve with 1 cup fresh pineapple slices (97).
TOTAL MEAL: 414 calories

Shrimp Jambalaya

■ PREP TIME: 15 MINUTES ■ TOTAL TIME: 50 MINUTES ■ MAKES 4 SERVINGS (1 CUP EACH)
■ MUFA: OLIVE OIL, GREEN OLIVES

Be sure to check the label on your Cajun seasoning for hidden sources of gluten. Or, blend your own, using our Cajun Spice Mix on page 66.

2 tablespoons olive oil

1 onion, chopped

1 red bell pepper, chopped

2 cloves garlic, chopped

1½ teaspoons gluten-free salt-free Cajun seasoning

¼ teaspoon salt

1 can (14½ ounces) no-salt-added stewed tomatoes

¼ cup quick-cooking brown rice

20 pimiento-stuffed green olives

¾ pound peeled and deveined medium shrimp

¼ cup chopped fresh parsley

Hot-pepper sauce (optional)

1. Preheat the oven to 375°F.

2. In a Dutch oven over medium-high heat, warm the oil. Add the onion, bell pepper, garlic, Cajun seasoning, and salt and cook, stirring occasionally, for 8 minutes, or until the vegetables are softened. Stir in the tomatoes, rice, and olives and bring to a boil. Cover and bake for 10 minutes.

3. Add the shrimp, tucking them into the sauce. Cover and bake for 5 to 6 minutes, or until the shrimp are opaque. Let stand for 10 minutes. Stir in the parsley right before serving and serve with the hot-pepper sauce at the table, if using.

Nutrition per serving: 264 calories, 19 g protein, 17 g carbohydrates, 13 g total fat, 1 g saturated fat, 3 g fiber, 718 mg sodium

Make It a
FLAT
BELLY
DIET
MEAL

Serve with 2 Lemon–Pine Nut Cookies (page 274) (144).
TOTAL MEAL: 408 calories

Tuna Noodle Casserole

■ PREP TIME: 15 MINUTES ■ TOTAL TIME: 50 MINUTES ■ MAKES 4 SERVINGS
■ MUFA: CANOLA OIL MAYONNAISE

If you prepare the noodles ahead of time, you can have this dish ready to pop in the oven as soon as the oven is finished preheating.

6 ounces gluten-free corn fusilli pasta

1 can (14 ounces) water-packed artichoke hearts, drained and chopped

1 can (5 ounces) water-packed chunk light tuna, drained

1 cup frozen peas

¼ cup canola oil mayonnaise

1 tablespoon grated lemon peel

1 tablespoon lemon juice

¼ cup grated Parmesan cheese, divided

6 gluten-free multigrain crackers, coarsely crushed

1. Preheat the oven to 350°F. Coat an 8″ x 8″ baking dish with cooking spray.

2. Prepare the pasta according to package directions. Drain.

3. In a large bowl, combine the artichoke hearts, tuna, peas, mayonnaise, lemon peel, lemon juice, and 2 tablespoons of the cheese. Toss gently to mix well. Stir in the pasta and spread evenly in the baking dish.

4. Scatter the crackers and the remaining 2 tablespoons cheese evenly over the top and bake for 30 to 35 minutes, or until the edges are bubbly and the top is golden.

Nutrition per serving: 323 calories, 17 g protein, 49 g carbohydrates, 7 g total fat, 1 g saturated fat, 9 g fiber, 717 mg sodium

Make It a FLAT BELLY DIET MEAL

Serve with 1 cup steamed broccoli (40) drizzled with 2 teaspoons trans-free margarine (54).
TOTAL MEAL: 417 calories

POULTRY

Curried Cashew Chicken

■ PREP TIME: 10 MINUTES ■ TOTAL TIME: 30 MINUTES ■ MAKES 4 SERVINGS ■ MUFA: CASHEWS

You'll be impressed by how a dish with so few ingredients can taste so complex.

1 cup packed fresh cilantro leaves
½ cup unsalted roasted cashews
1 tablespoon curry powder
1 cup gluten-free low-sodium chicken broth
¼ teaspoon salt

1 pound boneless, skinless chicken thighs, trimmed and cut into 2" pieces
1 cup frozen peas
2 tablespoons lime juice

1. In a food processor, combine the cilantro, cashews, and curry powder. Pulse to a paste. With the machine running, add the broth. The mixture will be runny and grainy.

2. Transfer the mixture to a medium nonstick skillet and add the salt. Bring to a simmer over medium heat. Tuck the chicken into the sauce and simmer, stirring occasionally, for 12 to 15 minutes, or until the chicken is cooked through and no longer pink. Stir in the peas and cook for 3 minutes, or until heated through.

3. Remove from the heat and stir in the lime juice.

Nutrition per serving: 294 calories, 26 g protein, 12 g carbohydrates, 16 g total fat, 3.5 g saturated fat, 2 g fiber, 275 mg sodium

Make It a
FLAT
BELLY
DIET
MEAL

Serve with ½ cup cooked brown rice (109).
TOTAL MEAL: 403 calories

Chicken and Broccoli with Peanut BBQ Sauce

■ PREP TIME: 15 MINUTES ■ TOTAL TIME: 35 MINUTES ■ MAKES 4 SERVINGS
■ MUFA: PEANUT BUTTER

You'll have no problem getting your family to finish their broccoli with this tangy peanut sauce served alongside.

1 pound boneless, skinless chicken breast, cut into 1" pieces
1 tablespoon fresh lime juice
1 teaspoon ground cumin
1 teaspoon paprika
1 clove garlic, minced
1/8 teaspoon salt
1/2 cup creamy natural unsalted peanut butter

1/3 cup gluten-free barbecue sauce
1 chipotle chile pepper in adobo sauce, finely chopped
5 tablespoons water, divided
1 tablespoon canola oil
4 cups broccoli florets
1 tablespoon fresh lemon juice

1. In a large bowl, toss the chicken, lime juice, cumin, paprika, garlic, and salt until well mixed. Let stand for 10 minutes.

2. Meanwhile, in a small bowl, whisk together the peanut butter, barbecue sauce, chile pepper, and 3 tablespoons of the water until smooth. Set aside.

3. In a large nonstick skillet over medium-high heat, warm the oil. Cook the chicken for 8 minutes, turning occasionally, or until browned and cooked through. Transfer to a plate and keep warm.

4. Wipe out the skillet. Reduce the heat to medium and add the broccoli and the remaining 2 tablespoons water. Cover and steam for 2 to 3 minutes, or until bright green and tender. Drizzle the lemon juice over the broccoli and toss to coat. Serve the chicken and broccoli with the sauce.

Nutrition per serving: 423 calories, 33 g protein, 21 g carbohydrates, 23 g total fat, 3 g saturated fat, 5 g fiber, 376 mg sodium

Make It a
FLAT
BELLY
DIET
MEAL

A single serving of this recipe counts as a Flat Belly Diet Meal without any add-ons!

Chicken Cobbler
with Cornmeal-Pepita Topping

■ PREP TIME: 20 MINUTES ■ TOTAL TIME: 1 HOUR 20 MINUTES ■ MAKES 6 SERVINGS
■ MUFA: PUMPKIN SEEDS, OLIVE OIL

Here's a new twist on what most people think of when it comes to comfort food. Roasted pumpkin seeds add MUFA power and a nutty texture to the topping.

FILLING

- 2 tablespoons olive oil
- 1 large leek, chopped
- 2 carrots, finely chopped
- 2 cups gluten-free low-sodium chicken broth
- 1/2 pound baby new potatoes, halved
- 2 cups cooked cubed chicken breast
- 3 tablespoons gluten-free all-purpose flour blend
- 3 tablespoons water
- 1 cup frozen peas
- 1/2 teaspoon salt

TOPPING

- 1 cup gluten-free all-purpose flour blend
- 1/2 cup gluten-free cornmeal
- 1/4 cup chopped roasted unsalted pumpkin seeds
- 1 teaspoon baking powder
- 1/2 teaspoon baking soda
- 1/2 teaspoon xanthan gum
- 3/4 cup buttermilk
- 1 egg
- 2 tablespoons olive oil

1. **To make the filling:** In a large saucepan, heat the oil over medium-high heat. Add the leek and carrots and cook, stirring occasionally, for 8 minutes, or until tender. Add the broth, potatoes, and chicken and bring to a boil. Reduce the heat to low, cover, and simmer for 10 minutes, or until the potatoes are almost tender.

2. In a small bowl, whisk together the flour and water until smooth. Stir into the saucepan and cook, stirring occasionally, for 15 minutes, or until the mixture bubbles and thickens. Stir in the peas and salt. Transfer the filling to a 1½-quart baking dish. Preheat the oven to 400°F.

3. **To make the topping:** In a large bowl, combine the flour, cornmeal, pumpkin seeds, baking powder, baking soda, and xanthan gum. In a small bowl, whisk together the buttermilk, egg, and oil. Add to the flour mixture, stirring to make a coarse-grained batter.

4. Drop the batter evenly over the filling. Place the baking dish on a small baking sheet to prevent drips. Bake for 25 minutes, or until the topping is golden and the filling is bubbly.

Nutrition per serving: 406 calories, 22 g protein, 43 g carbohydrates, 17 g total fat, 3 g saturated fat, 4 g fiber, 527 mg sodium

**Make It a
FLAT
BELLY
DIET
MEAL** } A single serving of this recipe counts as a Flat Belly Diet Meal without any add-ons!

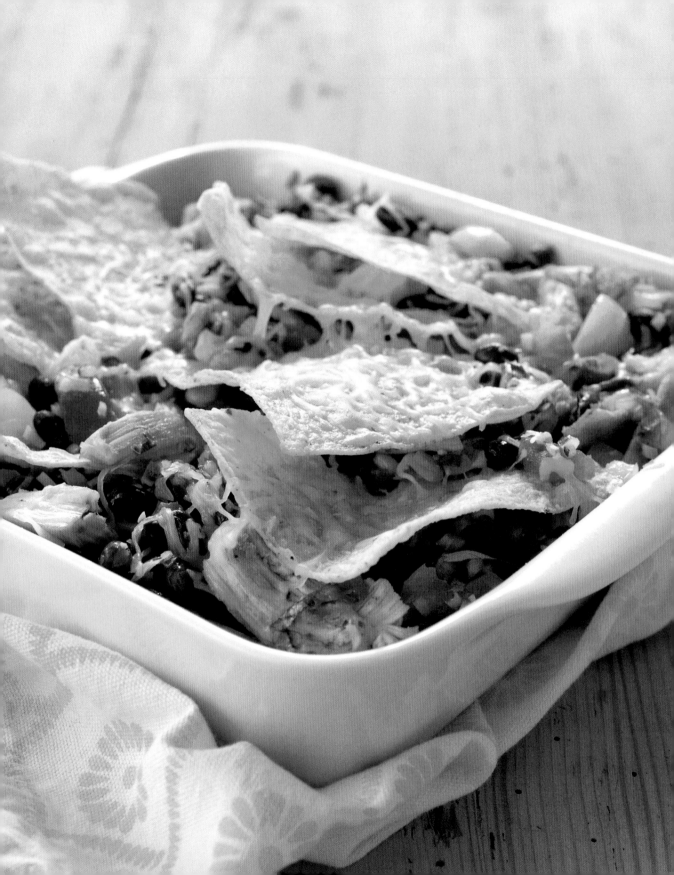

Fiesta Casserole

PREP TIME: 15 MINUTES ■ **TOTAL TIME: 45 MINUTES** ■ **MAKES 4 SERVINGS** ■ **MUFA: AVOCADO**

If you like, assemble this dish the night before you plan to serve it, then cover and refrigerate it. The next day, just pop it in the oven and you're done!

1 tablespoon olive oil	1/2 cup frozen corn kernels
1 onion, chopped	1/2 cup gluten-free black bean salsa
1 yellow bell pepper, chopped	2 ounces gluten-free corn tortilla chips, divided
1 tomato, chopped	
1 can (4 ounces) chopped mild green chiles, drained	1/2 cup shredded reduced-fat Mexican blend cheese, divided
2 cloves garlic, minced	1 Hass avocado, peeled, pitted, and cut into 16 slices
2 cups cooked cubed chicken breast	

1. Preheat the oven to 350°F. Coat an 8" x 8" baking dish with cooking spray.

2. In a large nonstick skillet over medium-high heat, warm the oil. Add the onion, bell pepper, tomato, chiles, and garlic and cook, stirring, for 5 minutes, or until softened. Stir in the chicken, corn, and salsa. Remove from the heat.

3. Line the bottom of the baking dish with half of the tortilla chips. Top with the chicken mixture, then sprinkle with 1/4 cup of the cheese. Coarsely crumble the remaining chips over the top. Sprinkle with the remaining 1/4 cup cheese. Transfer to the oven and bake for 20 minutes, or until the filling is hot and the cheese is melted. Let stand for 5 minutes before serving.

4. Cut into 4 servings and top each with 4 avocado slices.

Nutrition per serving: 393 calories, 31 g protein, 28 g carbohydrates, 18 g total fat, 4 g saturated fat, 6 g fiber, 467 mg sodium

Make It a
FLAT
BELLY
DIET
MEAL

A single serving of this recipe counts as a Flat Belly Diet Meal without any add-ons!

Broccoli-Chicken Casserole

■ PREP TIME: 10 MINUTES ■ TOTAL TIME: 1 HOUR ■ MAKES 4 SERVINGS ■ MUFA: ALMONDS

Chicken tenders are great to have on hand because they don't require much prepping. The convenience does make them a bit more expensive than boneless, skinless chicken breasts, so feel free to use those if you prefer.

1½ cups gluten-free low-sodium chicken broth

2 tablespoons cornstarch

1 tablespoon gluten-free Dijon mustard

1 tablespoon canola oil

1 pound boneless, skinless chicken tenders, cut into 1" chunks

1 onion, chopped

2 cups broccoli florets

1 cup instant brown rice

½ cup sliced almonds

½ cup shredded reduced-fat Cheddar cheese

1. Preheat the oven to 350°F. Coat an 8" x 8" baking dish with cooking spray.

2. In a medium bowl, whisk together the broth, cornstarch, and mustard until smooth. Set aside.

3. In a large nonstick skillet over medium-high heat, warm the oil. Add the chicken and onion and cook, stirring occasionally, for 5 minutes, or until browned. Add the reserved broth mixture and bring to a boil over medium-high heat. Reduce the heat to medium and cook, stirring often, for 2 minutes, or until the sauce is thickened. Remove from the heat and stir in the broccoli and rice.

4. Transfer the mixture to the baking dish and sprinkle the almonds and cheese evenly over the top. Cover loosely with a tent of foil and bake for 20 minutes. Uncover and bake for 10 minutes, or until the nuts are lightly browned and the cheese is melted. Let stand for 10 minutes before serving.

Nutrition per serving: 382 calories, 34 g protein, 28 g carbohydrates, 16 g total fat, 3 g saturated fat, 4 g fiber, 335 mg sodium

Make It a FLAT BELLY DIET MEAL } A single serving of this recipe counts as a Flat Belly Diet meal without any add-ons!

Turkey-Walnut Meat Loaf
with Mushroom Gravy

■ PREP TIME: 10 MINUTES ■ TOTAL TIME: 35 MINUTES ■ MAKES 4 SERVINGS ■ MUFA: WALNUTS

These individual meat loaves come together in considerably less time because they cook faster on the stove top than in the oven.

½ cup toasted walnuts	1 egg, lightly beaten
½ onion, coarsely chopped	½ teaspoon dried thyme
1 package (8 ounces) sliced cremini mushrooms, divided	½ teaspoon salt
1 pound ground turkey	1 teaspoon olive oil
¾ cup gluten-free rolled oats	¼ cup water
2 tablespoons ketchup	¼ cup 0% plain Greek yogurt

1. In a food processor, combine the walnuts, onion, and half of the mushrooms. Pulse five or six times, or until finely chopped. Transfer to a large bowl.

2. Add the turkey, oats, ketchup, egg, thyme, and salt. Gently mix to combine. Form into four 5" oblong loaves, about 1½" thick.

3. In a large nonstick skillet over medium-high heat, warm the oil. Add the loaves and cook for 4 minutes on each side, or until browned. Top with the remaining mushrooms and pour the water into the center of the skillet. Reduce the heat to low, cover, and cook for 15 minutes, or until a thermometer inserted in the center of a loaf registers 165°F. Transfer the loaves to a plate.

4. Stir the yogurt into the mushroom mixture in the skillet and remove from the heat. Serve the loaves with the sauce.

Nutrition per serving: 375 calories, 29 g protein, 19 g carbohydrates, 21 g fat, 4 g saturated fat, 3 g fiber, 519 mg sodium

Make It a
FLAT
BELLY
DIET
MEAL
} A single serving of this recipe counts as a Flat Belly Diet Meal without any add-ons!

Turkey Cutlets with Bacon and Avocado

■ PREP TIME: 10 MINUTES ■ TOTAL TIME: 20 MINUTES ■ MAKES 4 SERVINGS ■ MUFA: AVOCADO

With a high-quality hard-anodized nonstick skillet, you can brown turkey, chicken, or other cuts of meat in a small amount of oil. Here's how: Preheat the pan and add the oil, then spread with a silicone brush. Let it heat for 1 minute before adding the cutlets.

1 Hass avocado, peeled, pitted, and cubed	$\frac{1}{4}$ teaspoon ground black pepper, divided
1 tomato, chopped	4 boneless, skinless turkey cutlets (4 ounces each)
1 tablespoon chopped fresh cilantro	
2 teaspoons lime juice	1 teaspoon canola oil
$\frac{1}{4}$ teaspoon salt, divided	2 slices crisp-cooked gluten-free bacon, crumbled

1. In a medium bowl, mash the avocado with a fork. Add the tomato, cilantro, lime juice, $\frac{1}{8}$ teaspoon of the salt, and $\frac{1}{8}$ teaspoon of the pepper and stir until well mixed.

2. Cut each cutlet in half horizontally by slicing parallel to the work surface. Pound lightly to an even thickness between 2 sheets of plastic wrap. Season with the remaining $\frac{1}{8}$ teaspoon salt and $\frac{1}{8}$ teaspoon pepper.

3. In a large nonstick skillet over medium-high heat, warm the oil. Cook the cutlets for 3 to 4 minutes per side, or until browned and cooked through. Transfer to a platter. Top evenly with the avocado mixture and sprinkle with the bacon.

Nutrition per serving: 215 calories, 30 g protein, 5 g carbohydrates, 9 g total fat, 1.5 g saturated fat, 3 g fiber, 346 mg sodium

Make It a FLAT BELLY DIET MEAL

Serve with a Ginger-Blueberry Parfait (page 281), omitting the avocado (160).

TOTAL MEAL: 375 calories

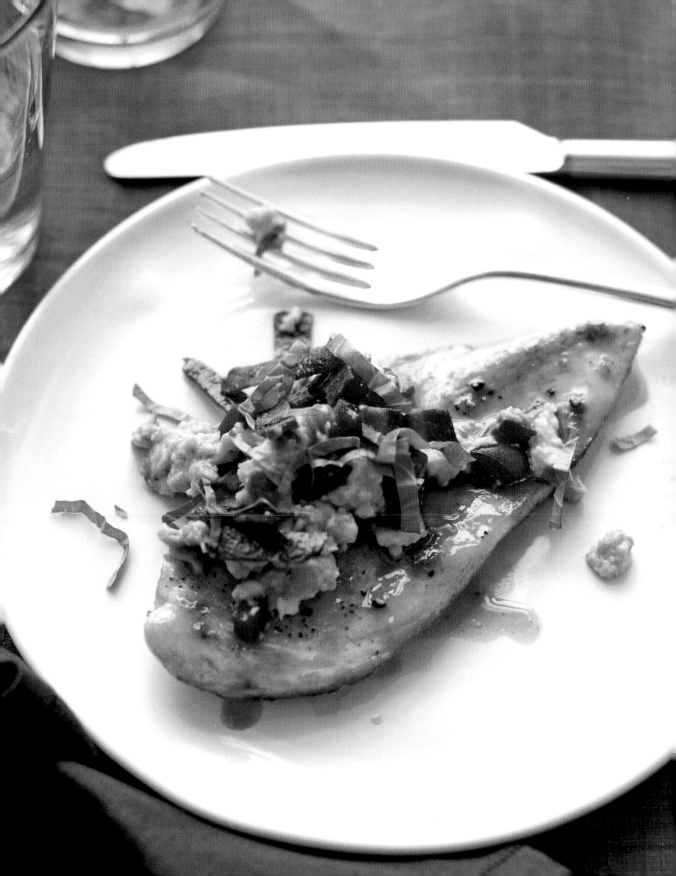

Grilled Sausage-Stuffed Zucchini Boats

■ PREP TIME: 15 MINUTES ■ TOTAL TIME: 1 HOUR 5 MINUTES ■ MAKES 4 SERVINGS ■ MUFA: OLIVES

This rustic vegetable dish has only a fraction of the saturated fat of a version made with pork sausage, thanks to the Italian turkey sausage in the stuffing. For a meatless version, use 3 ounces of Italian soy sausage instead.

1 link (3 ounces) Italian turkey sausage, casing removed

2 zucchini (½ pound each), halved lengthwise

1 tomato, chopped

40 black olives, pitted and chopped

1 shallot, thinly sliced

1 egg white, beaten

4 tablespoons shredded reduced-fat four-cheese Italian blend, divided

¼ teaspoon ground black pepper

1 teaspoon olive oil

1. Preheat the grill to medium. Coat a 12" x 12" sheet of heavy-duty foil with cooking spray.

2. Coat a medium nonstick skillet with cooking spray and set over medium-high heat. Add the sausage and cook for 5 minutes, breaking it up with a wooden spoon, or until browned.

3. Meanwhile, with a melon baller or spoon, scoop out the flesh of each zucchini, leaving about a ¼" shell. Finely chop the flesh and add it to the skillet along with the tomato, olives, and shallot. Cook over medium-high heat, stirring occasionally, for 10 minutes, or until the tomato is softened and any liquid has evaporated. Remove from the heat and let cool for 5 minutes. Stir in the egg white, 3 tablespoons of the cheese, and the pepper until well mixed.

4. Rub the oil all over the zucchini shells. Spoon the filling evenly into the shells and press in firmly. Sprinkle with the remaining 1 tablespoon cheese. Place the foil on the grill rack and set the zucchini on the foil over indirect heat. Grill, covered, for 25 to 30 minutes, or until the filling is hot and the zucchini are tender.

Nutrition per serving: 159 calories, 9 g protein, 11 g carbohydrates, 10 g total fat, 1.5 g saturated fat, 3 g fiber, 600 mg sodium

Make It a FLAT BELLY DIET MEAL Serve with Garlic Mashed Potatoes (page 226) (254).
TOTAL MEAL: 413 calories

Chipotle Turkey Chili

■ PREP TIME: 15 MINUTES ■ TOTAL TIME: 1 HOUR 20 MINUTES
■ MAKES 4 SERVINGS (1½ CUPS EACH) ■ MUFA: AVOCADO

If you prefer a vegetarian version, omit the turkey, increase the beans to 2 (15.5-ounce) cans, and add 1 cup of texturized soy protein. As some brands may contain hidden sources of gluten, be sure to check the label to make certain it is gluten free.

1 tablespoon olive oil	1 can (14½ ounces) no-salt-added diced tomatoes
1 onion, chopped	1 cup water
1 green bell pepper, chopped	½ teaspoon salt
2 cloves garlic, chopped	1 can (15.5 ounces) no-salt-added pinto beans, rinsed and drained
1 pound ground turkey breast	
1 chipotle chile pepper in adobo sauce, chopped + 2 tablespoons adobo sauce	¼ cup + 2 tablespoons chopped fresh cilantro
	1 Hass avocado, peeled, pitted, and chopped
3 tablespoons chili powder	
2 teaspoons ground cumin	2 tablespoons lime juice

1. In a large nonstick saucepan over medium-high heat, warm the oil. Add the onion, bell pepper, and garlic and cook, stirring occasionally, for 8 minutes, or until softened.

2. Add the turkey and cook, breaking it up with a wooden spoon, for 8 minutes, or until browned. Add the chile pepper, adobo sauce, chili powder, and cumin and cook for 1 minute. Add the tomatoes, water, and salt and bring to a boil. Reduce the heat to medium-low, cover, and simmer, stirring occasionally, for 45 minutes, or until the chili is thickened slightly and the flavors are blended. Add the beans and heat through. Remove from the heat and stir in the ¼ cup cilantro.

3. Meanwhile, in a medium bowl, combine the avocado, lime juice, and the 2 tablespoons cilantro and toss until well mixed.

4. Ladle the chili into each of 4 bowls. Top each serving with one-fourth of the avocado mixture.

Nutrition per serving: 314 calories, 34 g protein, 24 g carbohydrates, 11 g total fat, 1 g saturated fat, 8 g fiber, 405 mg sodium

Make It a FLAT BELLY DIET MEAL

Serve with 1 cup pitted sweet cherries (90).
TOTAL MEAL: 404 calories

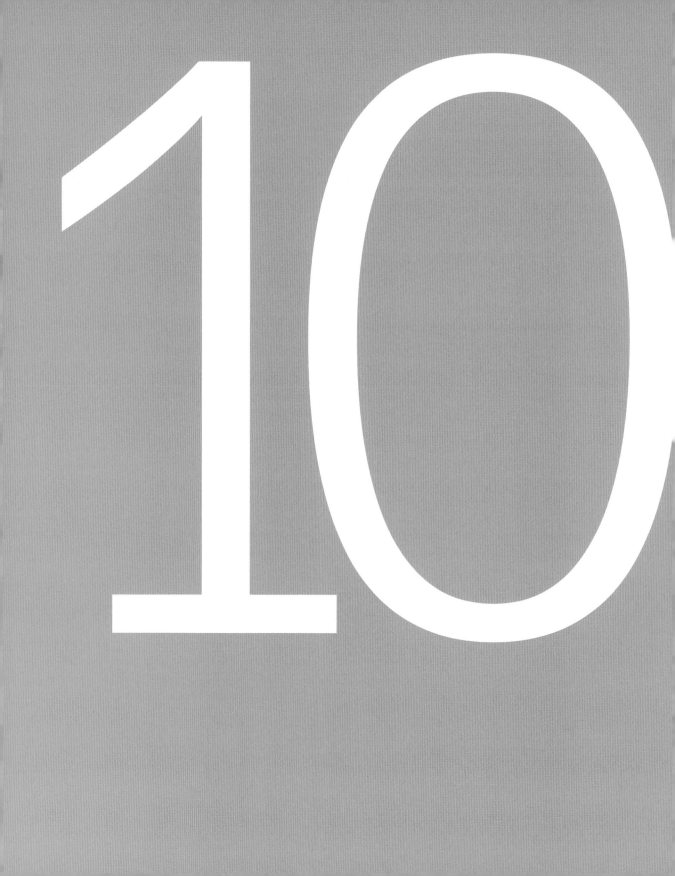

MEATS

Grilled Steak with Blue Cheese and Walnuts

■ PREP TIME: 10 MINUTES ■ TOTAL TIME: 25 MINUTES ■ MAKES 4 SERVINGS ■ MUFA: WALNUTS

Be sure to choose brands of blue cheese that are gluten free, like Maytag Blue and BelGioioso.

2 tablespoons red wine vinegar
1 tablespoon olive oil
1 tablespoon finely chopped shallot
¾ teaspoon salt, divided

¼ cup crumbled blue cheese
1 pound sirloin steak, trimmed of all visible fat
¼ teaspoon ground black pepper
½ cup toasted walnuts, chopped

1. In a small bowl, whisk together the vinegar, oil, shallot, and ¼ teaspoon of the salt until blended. Stir in the blue cheese and set aside.

2. Coat a grill rack or nonstick grill pan with cooking spray and preheat it to medium. Sprinkle the steak with the pepper and the remaining ½ teaspoon salt. Cook for 8 minutes, turning once, or until a thermometer inserted in the center registers 145°F for medium-rare. Let stand for 5 minutes before thinly slicing across the grain. Serve with the sauce and sprinkle with the walnuts.

Nutrition per serving: 343 calories, 27 g protein, 2 g carbohydrates, 25 g total fat, 7 g saturated fat, 1 g fiber, 613 mg sodium

Make It a FLAT BELLY DIET MEAL

Serve with 1 cup steamed asparagus (40).
TOTAL MEAL: 383 calories

Argentine-Style Grilled Steak with Chimichurri

■ PREP TIME: 10 MINUTES ■ TOTAL TIME: 25 MINUTES ■ MAKES 4 SERVINGS ■ MUFA: OLIVE OIL

Chimichurri sauce is the pesto of South America. Its bright green color and piquant flavors take an ordinary steak to new heights.

1/4 cup olive oil	2 cloves garlic, minced
1/4 cup chopped fresh parsley	1/2 teaspoon ground cumin
1/4 cup chopped fresh basil	1/4 teaspoon red-pepper flakes
3 tablespoons chopped fresh cilantro	1/2 teaspoon salt, divided
2 tablespoons lime juice	1 pound sirloin steak, trimmed of all visible fat
1 tablespoon red wine vinegar	

1. In a food processor, combine the oil, parsley, basil, cilantro, lime juice, vinegar, garlic, cumin, red-pepper flakes, and 1/4 teaspoon of the salt. Pulse to a puree. Set the chimichurri sauce aside.

2. Coat a grill rack or nonstick grill pan with cooking spray and preheat it to medium. Sprinkle the steak with the remaining 1/4 teaspoon salt. Grill the steak for 8 minutes, turning once, or until a thermometer inserted in the center registers 145°F for medium-rare. Let stand for 5 minutes before thinly slicing across the grain. Serve with the chimichurri sauce.

Nutrition per serving: 289 calories, 25 g protein, 2 g carbohydrates, 20 g total fat, 4.5 g saturated fat, 1 g fiber, 357 mg sodium

Make It a
FLAT
BELLY
DIET
MEAL
} Serve with 1 medium baked sweet potato without skin (103).
TOTAL MEAL: 392 calories

Olive-Stuffed Beef Rolls

■ PREP TIME: 20 MINUTES ■ TOTAL TIME: 35 MINUTES ■ MAKES 4 SERVINGS
■ MUFA: OLIVES, OLIVE OIL

Because it's so lean, top round can be a relatively bland cut of beef, but in this dish, it's practically bursting with flavor from the intense olive and tomato combination inside. Be careful not to overcook, as it will toughen considerably.

½ cup dry-packed sun-dried tomatoes	2 thin top round steaks, trimmed (¾ pound each)
20 kalamata olives, pitted	1 teaspoon + 2 tablespoons olive oil
2 cloves garlic, minced	2 tablespoons chopped fresh basil
1 teaspoon dried oregano	1 tablespoon lemon juice
¼ teaspoon ground black pepper	

1. In a food processor, combine the sun-dried tomatoes, olives, garlic, oregano, and pepper. Pulse until finely chopped.

2. Pound the meat to a ¼" thickness between 2 sheets of plastic wrap or waxed paper using a meat mallet or the bottom of a heavy skillet. With a sharp knife, lightly score the steaks on one side in a crosshatch pattern.

3. Evenly divide the filling between the 2 steaks, leaving a ½" border. Starting from the long side, roll up the steaks, jelly-roll fashion. Tie the rolls in 4 or 5 places with kitchen string.

4. In a large nonstick skillet over medium-high heat, warm the 1 teaspoon oil. Cook the rolls for 5 minutes, turning to brown on all sides. Transfer to a plate.

5. In a small bowl, combine the basil, lemon juice, and 2 tablespoons oil. Spoon evenly over the steaks. Let rest for 10 minutes before slicing into 1"-thick slices.

Nutrition per serving: 319 calories, 37 g protein, 7 g carbohydrates, 19 g total fat, 4 g saturated fat, 1 g fiber, 530 mg sodium

Make It a FLAT BELLY DIET MEAL

Serve with ½ cup cooked quinoa (111).
TOTAL MEAL: 430 calories

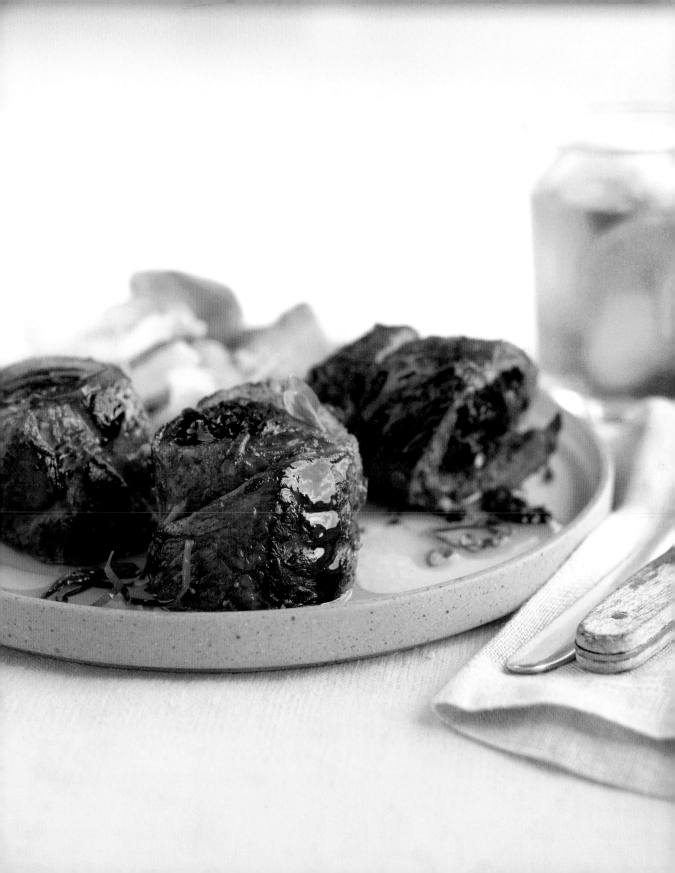

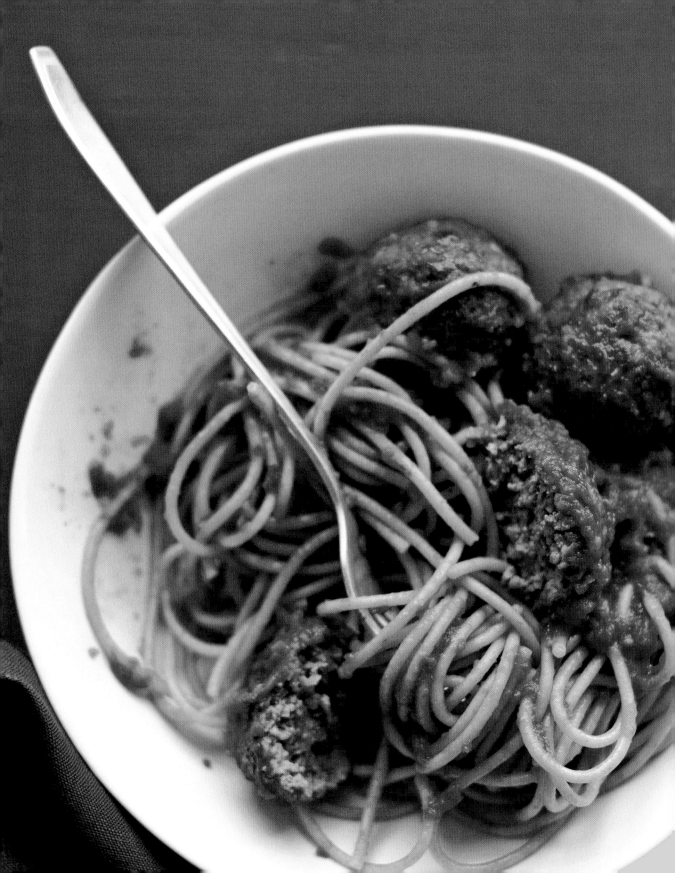

Family-Style Spaghetti and Meatballs

▓ PREP TIME: 20 MINUTES ▓ TOTAL TIME: 1 HOUR ▓ MAKES 8 SERVINGS ▓ MUFA: OLIVE OIL

Brown rice spaghetti is a good choice for this recipe. The texture holds up nicely, and it has a mild taste and nice bite. For a more authentic Italian flavor, use canned tomatoes from the San Marzano region of Italy.

1 slice gluten-free sandwich bread, torn into pieces	4 tablespoons olive oil, divided
1/4 cup fat-free milk	3 cloves garlic, minced
1 large egg	1 can (28 ounces) Italian peeled tomatoes
3/4 teaspoon salt, divided	1/4 cup chopped fresh basil
1 pound lean ground beef	1/4 teaspoon red-pepper flakes (optional)
1/4 cup grated Parmesan cheese	12 ounces gluten-free brown rice spaghetti or linguine
3 tablespoons chopped fresh parsley	

1. In a large bowl, combine the bread and milk and let stand for 5 minutes, or until the bread is softened and absorbs most of the milk. Stir in the egg and 1/2 teaspoon of the salt. Add the beef, cheese, and parsley and mix gently until combined. With lightly moistened hands, shape into 24 meatballs.

2. In a large nonstick skillet over medium-high heat, warm 1 1/2 teaspoons of the oil. Cook half of the meatballs for 5 to 7 minutes, turning occasionally, or until browned. Transfer to a plate and repeat with the remaining meatballs and 1 1/2 teaspoons of the oil.

3. Add the garlic and the remaining 3 tablespoons oil to the skillet and cook for 30 seconds, or until fragrant. Stir in the tomatoes, basil, red-pepper flakes (if using), and the remaining 1/4 teaspoon salt and bring to a boil. Reduce the heat and simmer for 5 minutes, or until the sauce thickens slightly.

4. Add the meatballs to the sauce in the skillet. Reduce the heat and simmer, partially covered, for 15 minutes, or until the flavors are blended and the meatballs are heated through.

5. Meanwhile, cook the spaghetti according to package directions. Serve the spaghetti topped with the sauce and meatballs.

Nutrition per serving: 350 calories, 19 g protein, 38 g carbohydrates, 12 g total fat, 3 g saturated fat, 2 g fiber, 536 mg sodium

Make It a FLAT BELLY DIET MEAL
Serve with 1 cup steamed green beans (44).
TOTAL MEAL: 394 calories

Beef Goulash Noodle Casserole

■ PREP TIME: 15 MINUTES ■ TOTAL TIME: 55 MINUTES ■ MAKES 4 SERVINGS ■ MUFA: CANOLA OIL

Baking this dish in the oven makes it easy to leave a meal cooking unattended. However, you could cook it on the stove, if you prefer. Just keep the lid on tight and turn the heat down to low.

¼ cup canola oil

1 onion, chopped

1 green bell pepper, chopped

2 teaspoons paprika

¾ pound lean ground beef

1 can (14.5 ounces) no-salt-added petite diced tomatoes

3 ounces gluten-free dried brown rice noodles

½ cup gluten-free low-sodium beef broth

¼ teaspoon salt

¼ cup reduced-fat sour cream

1 tablespoon gluten-free potato or tapioca starch

1. Preheat the oven to 350°F.

2. In a Dutch oven over medium-high heat, warm the oil. Add the onion, bell pepper, and paprika and cook, stirring occasionally, for 5 minutes, or until softened. Add the beef and cook, breaking it up with a wooden spoon, for 5 minutes, or until the beef is browned. Stir in the tomatoes, noodles, broth, and salt.

3. Cover tightly and bake for 15 minutes. Carefully remove the cover and stir. Return to the oven and bake, uncovered, for 10 minutes. Transfer to the stove top.

4. Whisk the sour cream and starch in a small bowl. Add to the casserole and place over medium-low heat. Stir for 1 to 2 minutes, or until thickened.

Nutrition per serving: 383 calories, 22 g protein, 30 g carbohydrates, 19 g total fat, 3 g saturated fat, 3 g fiber, 256 mg sodium

Make It a
FLAT
BELLY
DIET
MEAL

A single serving of this recipe counts as a Flat Belly Diet meal without any add-ons!

Lamb Koftas with Tomato Raita

■ PREP TIME: 20 MINUTES ■ TOTAL TIME: 30 MINUTES ■ MAKES 4 SERVINGS
■ MUFA: PINE NUTS, OLIVE OIL

Koftas are basically Middle Eastern meatballs. They are traditionally made with ground lamb, but you can use lean ground beef or even ground turkey, if you like.

1 tomato, chopped	1 pound lean ground lamb
½ cup 0% plain Greek yogurt	¼ cup pine nuts, chopped
2 tablespoons olive oil	2 tablespoons chopped fresh cilantro
2 tablespoons chopped fresh mint	2 cloves garlic, minced
1 tablespoon lemon juice	1 teaspoon ground cumin
½ teaspoon salt, divided	

1. In a medium bowl, combine the tomato, yogurt, oil, mint, lemon juice, and ¼ teaspoon of the salt until blended. Set the sauce aside.

2. In a large bowl, combine the lamb, pine nuts, cilantro, garlic, cumin, and the remaining ¼ teaspoon salt until well mixed. With damp hands, shape the lamb mixture into eight 4" oval shapes. Thread lengthwise onto eight 8" skewers, tapering the ends of each oval.

3. Coat a grill rack or nonstick grill pan with cooking spray and preheat it to medium. Grill the skewers for 8 minutes, turning occasionally, until the lamb is browned and cooked through. Serve with the sauce.

Nutrition per serving: 305 calories, 27 g protein, 5 g carbohydrates, 20 g total fat, 4.5 g saturated fat, 1 g fiber, 399 mg sodium

Make It a FLAT BELLY DIET MEAL
Serve with ½ cup brown rice (109).
TOTAL MEAL: 414 calories

Shish Kebabs with Lemon-Tahini Sauce

▓ PREP TIME: 15 MINUTES ▓ TOTAL TIME: 25 MINUTES ▓ MAKES 4 SERVINGS ▓ MUFA: TAHINI

**Store unused tahini in an airtight container in the refrigerator
for up to 3 months.**

3 tablespoons lemon juice, divided
2 teaspoons olive oil, divided
2 cloves garlic, minced
½ teaspoon dried oregano
1 pound pork loin, cut into 1" pieces

2 small zucchini, cut crosswise into 1" pieces
1 red bell pepper, cut into 1" pieces
½ red onion, quartered
¼ cup tahini
¼ cup water

1. In a large bowl, combine 2 tablespoons of the lemon juice, 1 teaspoon of the oil, the garlic, and oregano until blended. Add the pork, tossing to coat. Alternately thread the pork, zucchini, bell pepper, and onion on four 10" skewers.

2. Coat a grill rack or grill pan with cooking spray and preheat it to medium. Grill the skewers for 8 minutes, turning once, or until the pork is well marked and the vegetables are tender.

3. Meanwhile, in a small bowl, combine the tahini, water, and the remaining 1 tablespoon lemon juice and 1 teaspoon oil until blended. Drizzle each kebab with one-fourth of the sauce.

Nutrition per serving: 305 calories, 27 g protein, 10 g carbohydrates, 18 g total fat, 4 g saturated fat, 3 g fiber, 71 mg sodium

**Make It a
FLAT
BELLY
DIET
MEAL**

Serve with ½ cup cooked quinoa (111).
TOTAL MEAL: 416 calories

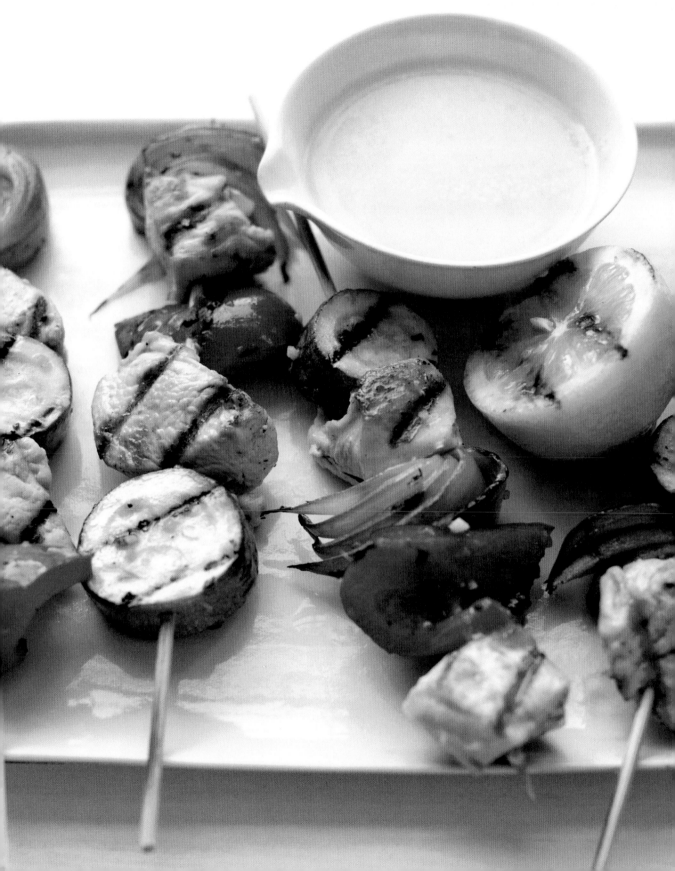

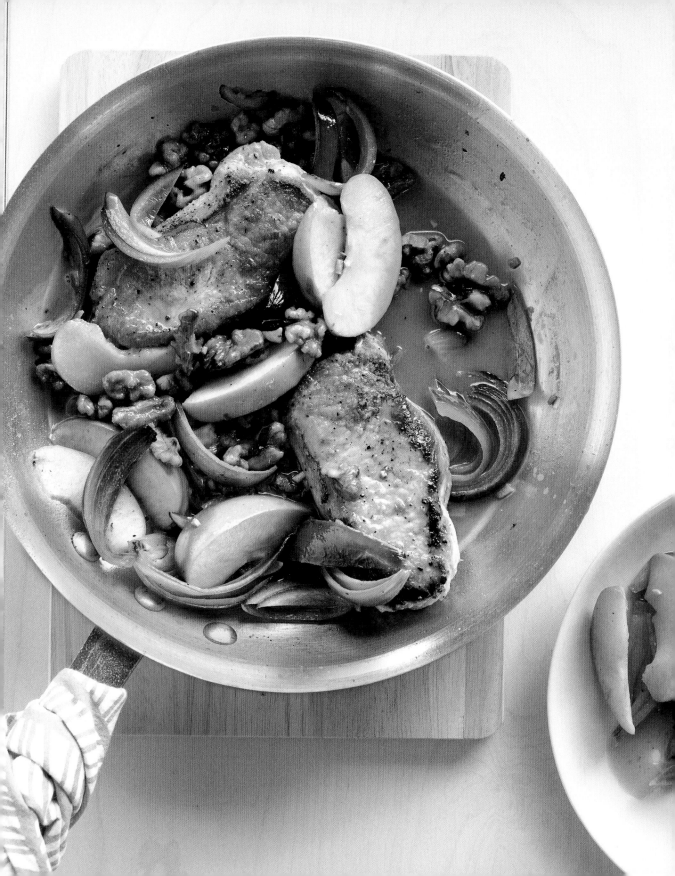

Cider Pork Chops
with Walnuts and Apples

■ PREP TIME: 10 MINUTES ■ TOTAL TIME: 35 MINUTES ■ MAKES 4 SERVINGS ■ MUFA: WALNUTS

A perfect skillet supper for fall—add a few dried prunes or dried apricots in with the apple mixture, if you like.

2 teaspoons canola oil, divided

4 boneless pork loin chops, trimmed (4 ounces each)

¼ teaspoon salt

¼ teaspoon ground black pepper

1 red onion, thinly sliced

1 Granny Smith apple, cored and sliced

2 cloves garlic, minced

½ cup apple cider

½ cup toasted walnuts, chopped

1. In a large nonstick skillet over medium-high heat, warm 1 teaspoon of the oil. Sprinkle the pork with the salt and pepper and cook for 6 minutes, turning once, or until browned. Transfer to a plate.

2. In the same skillet over medium-high heat, warm the remaining 1 teaspoon oil. Add the onion, apple, and garlic and cook, stirring occasionally, for 8 minutes, or until the onion and apple are softened. Add the cider and bring to a boil. Reduce the heat to medium and cook for 4 minutes, or until the cider is reduced by half. Return the pork (with any accumulated juices) to the skillet and cook for 3 minutes, or until a thermometer inserted in the center of a chop registers 160°F and the juices run clear.

3. Divide the pork among 4 plates. Top evenly with the onion-apple mixture and sprinkle 2 tablespoons of the walnuts over each serving.

Nutrition per serving: 292 calories, 28 g protein, 13 g carbohydrates, 14 g total fat, 2.5 g saturated fat, 2 g fiber, 206 mg sodium

Make It a
FLAT
BELLY
DIET
MEAL
Serve with 2 cups salad greens with 2 tablespoons balsamic vinaigrette (98).
TOTAL MEAL: 390 calories

Smoky Pork and Sweet Potato Skillet

■ PREP TIME: 20 MINUTES ■ TOTAL TIME: 40 MINUTES ■ MAKES 4 SERVINGS ■ MUFA: AVOCADO

You may find the heat in this dish to be a little intense. If so, substitute 1 tablespoon of your favorite mild chili powder in place of the chipotle. Just be sure it's gluten free.

1 Hass avocado, peeled, pitted, and cubed

1/4 cup chopped fresh cilantro

2 scallions, chopped

1/4 teaspoon salt

3/4 cup water, divided

3 tablespoons lime juice, divided

3 teaspoons olive oil, divided

1 pound pork tenderloin, trimmed and cut into 1" pieces

2 sweet potatoes, peeled and cut into 2" pieces

1 onion, finely chopped

2 teaspoons honey

1 chipotle chile pepper in adobo sauce, finely chopped

1. In a food processor, combine the avocado, cilantro, scallions, salt, 1/4 cup of the water, 2 tablespoons of the lime juice, and 2 teaspoons of the oil. Pulse for 30 seconds, or until smooth. Set aside.

2. Warm the remaining 1 teaspoon oil in a large nonstick skillet over medium-high heat. Cook the pork for 6 minutes, turning occasionally, or until browned. Transfer to a plate.

3. Add the potatoes, onion, and the remaining 1/2 cup water to the skillet. Reduce the heat to medium-low, cover, and cook, stirring occasionally, for 10 minutes, or until the potatoes are tender. Return the pork (with any accumulated juices) to the skillet. Add the honey, chile pepper, and the remaining 1 tablespoon lime juice to the skillet. Cook for 3 minutes, or until heated through.

4. Divide the pork mixture among 4 bowls and top each serving with one-fourth of the reserved avocado sauce.

Nutrition per serving: 290 calories, 26 g protein, 22 g carbohydrates, 11 g total fat, 2 g saturated fat, 5 g fiber, 266 mg sodium

Make It a
FLAT
BELLY
DIET
MEAL
} Serve with 1/2 serving of Garlicky Broccoli Rabe (page 221) (92).
TOTAL MEAL: 382 calories

Pork and Hominy Stew

■ PREP TIME: 15 MINUTES ■ TOTAL TIME: 50 MINUTES
■ MAKES 4 SERVINGS (1 ¼ CUPS EACH) ■ MUFA: AVOCADO

Hominy—the hulled corn kernels that have been stripped of the bran—is what gives this stew its unique taste. If you prefer, this is equally delicious with 1 can (15½ ounces) of black beans instead. Be sure to rinse and drain them first.

4 teaspoons olive oil, divided

1 pound lean pork tenderloin, cut into ¾" pieces

1 onion, chopped

1 carrot, chopped

1 rib celery, chopped

3 cloves garlic, chopped

1 teaspoon ground cumin

2 cups gluten-free low-sodium chicken broth

1 can (15 ounces) white hominy, rinsed and drained

2 plum tomatoes, chopped

3 tablespoons chopped fresh cilantro

½ teaspoon salt

1 Hass avocado, peeled, pitted, and cubed

¼ cup reduced-fat sour cream

1. In a Dutch oven over medium-high heat, warm 2 teaspoons of the oil. Cook the pork for 6 minutes, turning occasionally, or until lightly browned. Transfer to a plate and set aside.

2. Add the remaining 2 teaspoons oil to the Dutch oven. Add the onion, carrot, celery, garlic, and cumin and cook over medium heat, stirring occasionally, for 6 to 7 minutes, or until softened. Add the broth, hominy, and reserved pork. Bring to a boil over high heat. Reduce the heat to low, cover, and simmer for 20 minutes, or until the pork is tender. Stir in the tomatoes, cilantro, and salt.

3. In a small bowl, coarsely mash the avocado with the sour cream until well mixed. Divide the stew among 4 bowls and top each bowl with one-fourth of the avocado cream.

Nutrition per serving: 317 calories, 28 g protein, 17 g carbohydrates, 15 g total fat, 3.5 g saturated fat, 5 g fiber, 512 mg sodium

Make It a FLAT BELLY DIET MEAL

Serve with a medium apple (95).
TOTAL MEAL: 412 calories

SIDE DISHES

Roasted Carrots with Walnuts and Leeks

This lovely autumn side dish is satisfying and simple enough to prepare for the holiday table.

1 pound baby carrots	2 teaspoons balsamic vinegar
2 large leeks, white and light green parts only, cut lengthwise in half	¼ teaspoon salt
1 tablespoon olive oil	½ cup walnuts

1. Preheat the oven to 400°F. Coat a rimmed baking sheet with cooking spray.

2. In the pan, toss the carrots and leeks with the oil, vinegar, and salt. Spread the vegetables evenly in the baking sheet. Roast for 20 minutes.

3. Scatter the walnuts over the vegetables and roast for 10 minutes, or until the walnuts are golden and the vegetables are tender and lightly browned.

Nutrition per serving: 194 calories, 4 g protein, 20 g carbohydrates, 12 g total fat, 1 g saturated fat, 4 g fiber, 215 mg sodium

Make It a FLAT BELLY DIET MEAL

Serve with 3 ounces roast turkey (145) and ½ cup roasted baby red potatoes (75).

TOTAL MEAL: 414 calories

Zucchini Ribbons with Pine Nuts and Dill

■ PREP TIME: 15 MINUTES ■ TOTAL TIME: 15 MINUTES ■ MAKES 4 SERVINGS
■ MUFA: PINE NUTS, OLIVE OIL

Make this up to 1 hour ahead of time, to allow the flavors to fully develop.

3 medium zucchini

2 tablespoons extra-virgin olive oil

¼ cup toasted pine nuts

3 tablespoons chopped fresh dill

2 tablespoons lemon juice

¼ teaspoon salt

1. With a vegetable peeler, shave the zucchini into thin lengthwise slices. Transfer to a large bowl.

2. Add the oil, pine nuts, dill, lemon juice, and salt. Toss gently to combine.

Nutrition per serving: 146 calories, 3 g protein, 7 g carbohydrates, 13 g total fat, 1.5 g saturated fat, 2 g fiber, 160 mg sodium

Make It a
FLAT
BELLY
DIET
MEAL
} Serve with 3 ounces roasted pork tenderloin (122) and ½ cup cooked brown rice (109).
TOTAL MEAL: 377 calories

Asparagus-Sesame Stir-Fry

▦ PREP TIME: 10 MINUTES ▦ TOTAL TIME: 15 MINUTES ▦ MAKES 4 SERVINGS ▦ MUFA: CANOLA OIL

Asparagus are best when cooked briefly to retain the crispness. If you like, add a teaspoon of toasted sesame oil to the finished dish.

¼ cup canola oil
1 red bell pepper, cut into thin strips
1 pound asparagus, trimmed and cut into 2" pieces
1 tablespoon chopped peeled fresh ginger

1 tablespoon gluten-free reduced-sodium soy sauce
⅛ teaspoon red-pepper flakes
½ teaspoon toasted sesame seeds

1. In a large nonstick skillet over medium-high heat, warm the oil. Cook the bell pepper, stirring frequently, for 3 minutes, or until tender-crisp. Add the asparagus, ginger, soy sauce, and red-pepper flakes and cook for 2 minutes, or until heated through.

2. Remove from the heat and stir in the sesame seeds.

Nutrition per serving: 160 calories, 3 g protein, 7 g carbohydrates, 14 g total fat, 1 g saturated fat, 3 g fiber, 156 mg sodium

**Make It a
FLAT
BELLY
DIET
MEAL**

Serve with Grilled Steak with Blue Cheese and Walnuts (page 198), omitting the walnuts (261).
TOTAL MEAL: 421 calories

Roasted Brussels Sprouts with Hazelnuts

■ PREP TIME: 10 MINUTES ■ TOTAL TIME: 40 MINUTES ■ MAKES 4 SERVINGS ■ MUFA: HAZELNUTS

High-heat roasting is by far the best way to cook Brussels sprouts. They caramelize while roasting, which brings out all the natural sweetness.

1 pound Brussels sprouts, trimmed and halved lengthwise

1 sweet onion, cut into 8 wedges

½ cup skinned hazelnuts, coarsely chopped

1 tablespoon olive oil

½ teaspoon salt

¼ teaspoon ground black pepper

1. Preheat the oven to 450°F. Coat a rimmed baking sheet with cooking spray. On the baking sheet, toss the Brussels sprouts with the onion, hazelnuts, oil, salt, and pepper. Spread the vegetables evenly in the pan.

2. Roast, stirring occasionally, for 25 to 30 minutes, or until the Brussels sprouts are crisp and browned.

Nutrition per serving: 207 calories, 7 g protein, 18 g carbohydrates, 14 g total fat, 1.5 g saturated fat, 6 g fiber, 323 mg sodium

Make It a
FLAT
BELLY
DIET
MEAL
}
Serve with 3 ounces roasted chicken breast (140) and ½ cup grilled baby red potatoes (75).
TOTAL MEAL: 422 calories

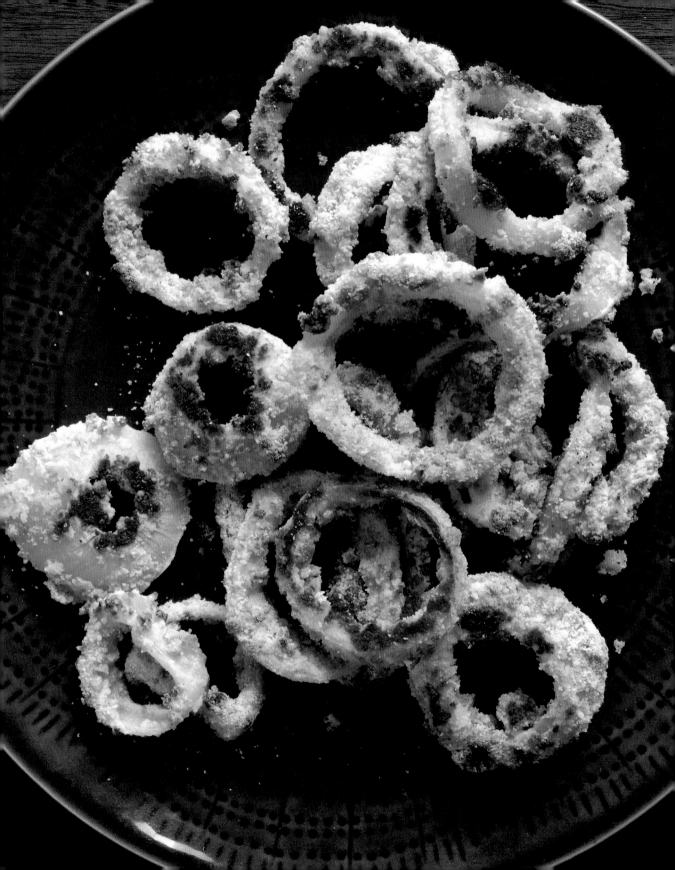

Onion Rings

■ PREP TIME: 10 MINUTES ■ TOTAL TIME: 30 MINUTES ■ MAKES 4 SERVINGS
■ MUFA: ALMOND MEAL

Serve these crunchy rings with your favorite mild or medium salsa.

1 large sweet onion, cut crosswise into ½"-thick rounds

⅓ cup gluten-free all-purpose flour

¼ teaspoon xanthan gum

½ cup low-fat buttermilk

1 egg white

1 cup gluten-free cornflakes, finely crushed

1 cup almond meal

½ teaspoon salt

1. Preheat the oven to 450°F. Coat 2 large baking sheets with cooking spray.

2. Separate the onion rounds into 16 rings. Place the flour and xanthan gum in a large resealable food storage bag. Add the onion rings, a few at a time. Seal the bag and shake until evenly coated.

3. In a medium bowl, whisk together the buttermilk and egg white until blended. Combine the crushed cornflakes, almond meal, and salt on a sheet of waxed paper. Dip the rings, one at a time, into the buttermilk mixture, then into the almond meal mixture. Transfer the rings to the baking sheets and lightly coat them with cooking spray.

4. Bake for 15 to 18 minutes, or until the onion rings are golden and crisp.

Nutrition per serving: 269 calories, 10 g protein, 29 g carbohydrates, 15 g total fat, 1 g saturated fat, 5 g fiber, 368 mg sodium

Make It a FLAT BELLY DIET MEAL

Serve with 1 turkey burger patty (150).
TOTAL MEAL: 419 calories

Creamy Sesame Collard Greens

■ PREP TIME: 10 MINUTES ■ TOTAL TIME: 35 MINUTES ■ MAKES 4 SERVINGS ■ MUFA: TAHINI

Old-school creamed spinach is drenched in a heavy cream-laden sauce. This MUFA-improved version uses collard greens instead of spinach and heart-healthy sesame paste to create a rich sauce.

1 teaspoon canola oil	$\frac{1}{2}$ cup water, divided
1 onion, chopped	$\frac{1}{2}$ cup tahini
1 large bunch collard greens (about 1$\frac{1}{2}$ pounds), tough stems removed, leaves coarsely chopped	1 tablespoon honey
	$\frac{1}{4}$ teaspoon salt
	$\frac{1}{8}$ teaspoon ground red pepper

1. In a large nonstick skillet over medium-high heat, warm the oil. Cook the onion, stirring occasionally, for 5 minutes, or until softened.

2. Add the collards, a few handfuls at a time, stirring and allowing the leaves to wilt before adding more. Add $\frac{1}{4}$ cup of the water and bring to a boil. Reduce the heat to medium-low, cover, and simmer, stirring occasionally, for 15 minutes, or until the collards are tender.

3. Meanwhile, in a small bowl, whisk together the tahini, honey, salt, red pepper, and the remaining $\frac{1}{4}$ cup water until smooth. Stir into the collard mixture and cook for 1 minute, or until heated through.

Nutrition per serving: 245 calories, 8 g protein, 19 g carbohydrates, 18 g total fat, 2.5 g saturated fat, 7 g fiber, 202 mg sodium

Make It a
FLAT
BELLY
DIET
MEAL

Serve with 3 ounces roasted pork tenderloin (122) and 1 cup chopped watermelon (40).
TOTAL MEAL: 407 calories

Garlicky Broccoli Rabe

■ PREP TIME: 10 MINUTES ■ TOTAL TIME: 20 MINUTES ■ MAKES 4 SERVINGS ■ MUFA: OLIVE OIL

If the natural bitterness of this green is unappealing, use 4 cups broccoli or cauliflower florets instead.

2 bunches broccoli rabe (about 2 pounds), tough stem ends removed

¼ cup extra-virgin olive oil

6 cloves garlic, thinly sliced

¼ teaspoon crushed red-pepper flakes

½ teaspoon salt

1. In a large skillet, bring 2" of water to a boil over high heat. Add the broccoli rabe, reduce the heat to medium, cover, and simmer for 3 minutes, or until tender-crisp. Drain well. Wipe the skillet dry.

2. In the same skillet, warm the oil over medium-high heat. Cook the garlic, stirring, for 2 minutes, or until lightly browned and fragrant. Add the broccoli rabe, red-pepper flakes, and salt and cook, stirring, for 2 minutes, or until heated through.

Nutrition per serving: 183 calories, 7 g protein, 8 g carbohydrates, 15 g total fat, 2 g saturated fat, 6 g fiber, 291 mg sodium

Make It a FLAT BELLY DIET MEAL

Serve with 4 pieces fried tofu (141) and 1 cup cooked shirataki noodles (53).

TOTAL MEAL: 377 calories

Roasted Peppers with Olives and Goat Cheese

■ PREP TIME: 10 MINUTES ■ TOTAL TIME: 30 MINUTES ■ MAKES 4 SERVINGS
■ MUFA: OLIVES, OLIVE OIL

This lively dish goes with just about everything. If you prefer to broil the peppers, line a broiler-pan rack with foil and coat it with cooking spray. Broil the peppers, skin side up, 4" from the heat, for 10 to 12 minutes, or until the skin is charred in spots.

4 large red, yellow, or green bell peppers, each cut lengthwise into 4 panels
2 tablespoons extra-virgin olive oil
¼ cup chopped fresh basil

20 oil-cured black olives, pitted and coarsely chopped
2 tablespoons reduced-fat goat cheese, crumbled

1. Coat a grill rack with cooking spray and preheat the grill to medium-high. Grill the peppers for 10 to 12 minutes, turning occasionally, or until the peppers are softened and charred in spots. Transfer to a work surface and let cool.

2. When cool enough to handle, peel the peppers and place them on a large plate. Drizzle with the oil, turning to coat. Top with the basil and olives, and sprinkle with the goat cheese.

Nutrition per serving: 139 calories, 3 g protein, 12 g carbohydrates, 10 g total fat, 1 g saturated fat, 3 g fiber, 172 mg sodium

Make It a
FLAT
BELLY
DIET
MEAL

Serve with 4 ounces thinly sliced broiled flank steak (218) and 1 clementine (35).
TOTAL MEAL: 392 calories

Slow-Roasted Tomatoes with Tapenade

▒ PREP TIME: 10 MINUTES ▒ TOTAL TIME: 1 HOUR 10 MINUTES ▒ MAKES 4 SERVINGS
▒ MUFA: BLACK OLIVE TAPENADE

Plum or Roma tomatoes work best with this simple technique because they have a firm, meaty texture, and fewer seeds than beefsteaks.

12 plum tomatoes, halved lengthwise

1 tablespoon olive oil

½ cup Black Olive Tapenade (page 80) or store-bought gluten-free tapenade

1. Preheat the oven to 325°F. Coat a rimmed baking sheet with cooking spray. On the baking sheet, toss the tomatoes with the oil until well coated. Spread the tomatoes evenly in the pan and roast for 50 to 60 minutes, or until the tomatoes are very soft but still hold their shape.

2. Transfer the tomatoes to a platter and top each with 1 teaspoon of the tapenade. Serve warm or at room temperature.

Nutrition per serving: 111 calories, 2 g protein, 9 g carbohydrates, 9 g total fat, 1 g saturated fat, 3 g fiber, 223 mg sodium

Make It a FLAT BELLY DIET MEAL
Serve with 3 ounces roast chicken breast (140), cut into strips, and laid over Caramelized Onion and Olive Focaccia (page 252), omitting the olives (166).
TOTAL MEAL: 417 calories

Chipotle and Brown Sugar Roasted Sweet Potatoes

■ PREP TIME: 10 MINUTES ■ TOTAL TIME: 40 MINUTES ■ MAKES 4 SERVINGS ■ MUFA: OLIVE OIL

Forget the traditional sweet potato casserole! The spicy-sweet combination of this dish will liven up any holiday menu.

2 sweet potatoes (about 1 pound), cut lengthwise into 8 wedges each	2 teaspoons gluten-free chipotle chili powder
¼ cup olive oil	½ teaspoon ground cumin
1 tablespoon packed light brown sugar	¼ teaspoon salt

1. Preheat the oven to 425°F.

2. Coat a rimmed baking sheet with cooking spray. On the baking sheet, toss the potatoes with the oil, brown sugar, chili powder, cumin, and salt. Spread the potatoes evenly in the pan and roast for 15 minutes. Turn the potatoes and roast for 15 minutes longer, or until golden brown and crisp.

Nutrition per serving: 231 calories, 2 g protein, 26 g carbohydrates, 14 g total fat, 2 g saturated fat, 3 g fiber, 209 mg sodium

Make It a
FLAT BELLY DIET MEAL

Serve with 3 ounces roast chicken breast (140) and 1 cup steamed broccoli (44).
TOTAL MEAL: 415 calories

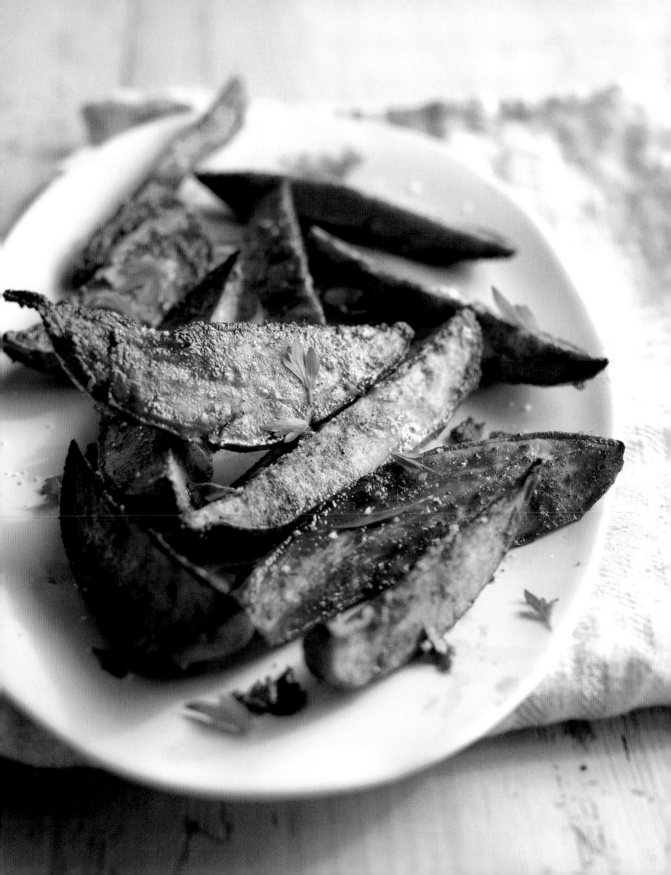

Garlic Mashed Potatoes

■ PREP TIME: 15 MINUTES ■ TOTAL TIME: 30 MINUTES ■ MAKES 4 SERVINGS ■ MUFA: OLIVE OIL

For even more fiber, scrub your potatoes well, but keep the skin on. Russet potatoes, also known as Idaho or baking potatoes, have a low moisture content, making them especially fluffy when cooked.

1½ pounds russet potatoes, cut into 2" pieces

4 whole cloves garlic

¼ cup olive oil

2 tablespoons 0% plain Greek yogurt

1 tablespoon chopped fresh chives

½ teaspoon salt

1. In a large saucepan, combine the potatoes, garlic, and enough water to cover by 2". Bring to a boil over high heat. Reduce the heat to medium-low, cover, and simmer for 15 minutes, or until tender. Drain and return to the pot.

2. Add the oil, yogurt, chives, and salt and mash with a potato masher until smooth.

Nutrition per serving: 254 calories, 4 g protein, 31 g carbohydrates, 14 g total fat, 2 g saturated fat, 2 g fiber, 294 mg sodium

Make It a
FLAT
BELLY
DIET
MEAL

Serve with 3 ounces roasted pork tenderloin (122) and ½ cup cooked spinach (21).
TOTAL MEAL: 397 calories

Orange-Pecan Rice with Cranberries

■ PREP TIME: 10 MINUTES ■ TOTAL TIME: 1 HOUR ■ MAKES 4 SERVINGS ■ MUFA: PECANS

You may substitute chicken broth for the water, if you prefer—just leave out the salt.

1 tablespoon olive oil
1 shallot, thinly sliced
2 cups water
¾ cup brown basmati rice
½ teaspoon salt

½ cup toasted pecans, coarsely chopped
½ cup dried cranberries
2 teaspoons grated orange peel

1. In a medium saucepan over medium-high heat, warm the oil. Cook the shallot, stirring occasionally, for 3 minutes, or until softened.

2. Add the water, rice, and salt and bring to a boil. Reduce the heat to medium-low, cover, and simmer for 40 to 45 minutes, or until the liquid is absorbed and the rice is tender. Fluff the rice with a fork and stir in the pecans, cranberries, and orange peel.

Nutrition per serving: 307 calories, 5 g protein, 42 g carbohydrates, 15 g total fat, 2 g saturated fat, 4 g fiber, 298 mg sodium

Make It a FLAT BELLY DIET MEAL
Serve with 2 ounces roast turkey (96).
TOTAL MEAL: 403 calories

Almond-Saffron Rice

■ PREP TIME: 5 MINUTES ■ TOTAL TIME: 35 MINUTES ■ MAKES 4 SERVINGS ■ MUFA: ALMONDS

Studded with slivers of toasted almonds, this fragrant rice makes a lovely side dish. Instant brown rice gets this on the table in under 30 minutes. If you have more time, prepare this dish with brown basmati rice instead.

½ teaspoon saffron threads	½ teaspoon salt
1 tablespoon + 2¼ cups water	1½ cups instant brown rice
1 teaspoon olive oil	½ cup slivered almonds, toasted

1. In a small bowl, soak the saffron in 1 tablespoon water for 20 minutes. Use the back of a spoon to mash the threads.

2. In a large saucepan, bring the oil, salt, and 2¼ cups water to a boil over high heat. Add the rice and the saffron mixture. Reduce the heat to low, cover, and simmer for 5 minutes. Turn off the heat and let the rice stand for 5 minutes.

3. Fluff the rice with a fork and stir in the almonds.

Nutrition per serving: 215 calories, 6 g protein, 28 g carbohydrates, 9 g total fat, 0.5 g saturated fat, 3 g fiber, 304 mg sodium

Make It a
FLAT
BELLY
DIET
MEAL

Serve with 3 ounces baked or broiled tilapia (145) and 1 cup steamed broccoli (44).
TOTAL MEAL: 404 calories

Fruity Millet Pilaf

■ PREP TIME: 10 MINUTES ■ TOTAL TIME: 45 MINUTES ■ MAKES 4 SERVINGS ■ MUFA: ALMONDS

This side dish is a great accompaniment to grilled lamb or chicken kebabs. Dried apples, raisins, or figs can be used in place of the apricots and dates.

2 teaspoons canola oil	1/4 teaspoon salt
2 scallions, thinly sliced	1/2 cup sliced almonds, toasted
2 1/4 cups water	1/4 cup dried apricots, chopped
2/3 cup millet	1/4 cup pitted chopped dates
1/4 cup orange juice	

1. In a large nonstick skillet over medium-high heat, warm the oil. Cook the scallions, stirring frequently, for 2 to 3 minutes, or until softened.

2. Add the water, millet, orange juice, and salt and bring to a boil. Reduce the heat to medium-low, cover, and simmer for 25 to 30 minutes, or until the millet is tender. Remove from the heat. Fluff the millet with a fork and stir in the almonds, apricots, and dates.

Nutrition per serving: 267 calories, 7 g protein, 41 g carbohydrates, 10 g total fat, 1 g saturated fat, 6 g fiber, 155 mg sodium

Make It a FLAT BELLY DIET MEAL
Serve with Lamb Koftas with Tomato Raita (page 205), omitting the Tomato Raita and pine nuts (165).
TOTAL MEAL: 432 calories

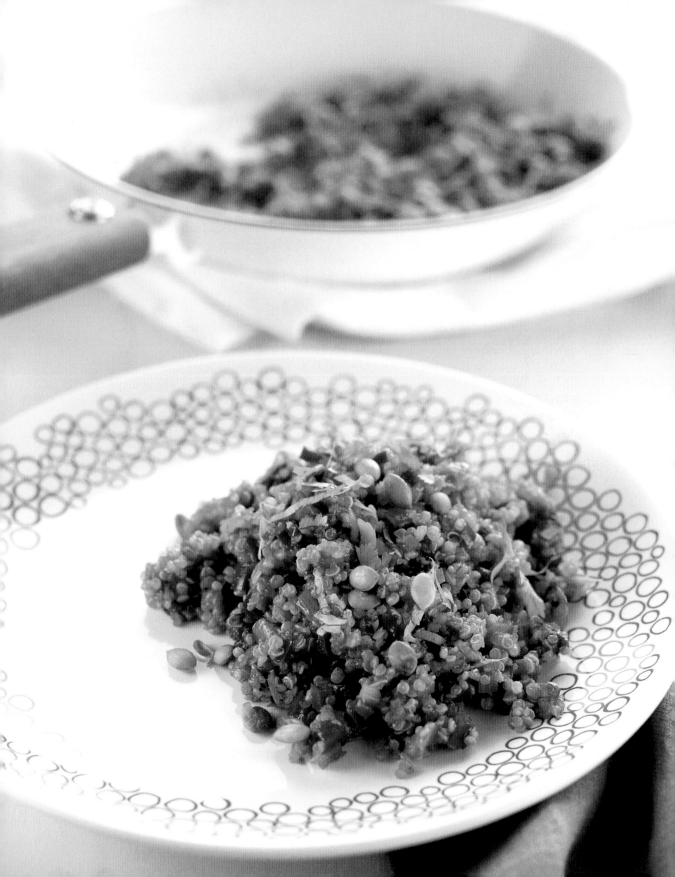

Tex-Mex-Style Quinoa

■ PREP TIME: 10 MINUTES ■ TOTAL TIME: 35 MINUTES ■ MAKES 4 SERVINGS
■ MUFA: PUMPKIN SEEDS

Make this a main dish by adding 2 cups cooked cubed tofu or chicken to this Tex-Mex-style stir-fry.

1 tablespoon olive oil	1 cup gluten-free low-sodium vegetable broth
1 onion, finely chopped	½ cup quinoa
1 red bell pepper, finely chopped	½ cup unsalted toasted pumpkin seeds
1 clove garlic, minced	2 tablespoons chopped fresh cilantro
1 teaspoon ground cumin	
¾ teaspoon chili powder	

1. In a large nonstick skillet over medium-high heat, warm the oil. Cook the onion and bell pepper, stirring occasionally, for 8 minutes, or until softened. Add the garlic, cumin, and chili powder and cook, stirring, for 1 minute, or until fragrant.

2. Add the broth and quinoa and bring to a boil. Reduce the heat, cover, and simmer for 15 minutes, or until the liquid is evaporated and the quinoa is tender. Remove from the heat. Fluff the quinoa with a fork and stir in the pumpkin seeds and cilantro.

Nutrition per serving: 221 calories, 8 g protein, 21 g carbohydrates, 12 g total fat, 2 g saturated fat, 4 g fiber, 42 mg sodium

Make It a
FLAT
BELLY
DIET
MEAL

Serve with 3 ounces roasted chicken breast (140) topped with 2 tablespoons gluten-free barbecue sauce (40).
TOTAL MEAL: 401 calories

Shirataki Noodles
with Mushrooms and Artichokes

▥ PREP TIME: 10 MINUTES ▥ TOTAL TIME: 25 MINUTES ▥ MAKES 4 SERVINGS
▥ MUFA: BLACK OLIVE TAPENADE, OLIVE OIL

Shirataki noodles are a great gluten-free substitute for wheat noodles. They are thin, low-calorie, low-carb, translucent Japanese noodles. You can find them in the refrigerated section of Asian markets, health food stores, and most supermarkets.

1 package (8 ounces) tofu shirataki noodles

2 tablespoons extra-virgin olive oil

1 package (8 ounces) sliced mushrooms

1 onion, chopped

3 cloves garlic, minced

1 pint cherry tomatoes

1 can (14 ounces) water-packed artichoke hearts, rinsed, drained, and chopped

¼ cup Black Olive Tapenade (page 80) or store-bought gluten-free tapenade

4 teaspoons grated Parmesan cheese

1. Prepare the noodles according to package directions. Drain.

2. Meanwhile, in a large nonstick skillet over medium-high heat, warm the oil. Cook the mushrooms and onion, stirring occasionally, for 8 minutes, or until tender. Add the garlic and cook for 1 minute. Stir in the tomatoes and artichokes and cook for 3 minutes, or until the tomatoes just begin to soften.

3. Add the noodles and heat through. Remove from the heat and stir in the tapenade.

4. Divide the noodle mixture among 4 bowls and top each with 1 teaspoon of the cheese.

Nutrition per serving: 186 calories, 6 g protein, 19 g carbohydrates, 11 g total fat, 1.5 g saturated fat, 6 g fiber, 612 mg sodium

Make It a
FLAT
BELLY
DIET
MEAL

Serve with 4 pieces fried tofu (141) and 2 medium plums (60).
TOTAL MEAL: 387 calories

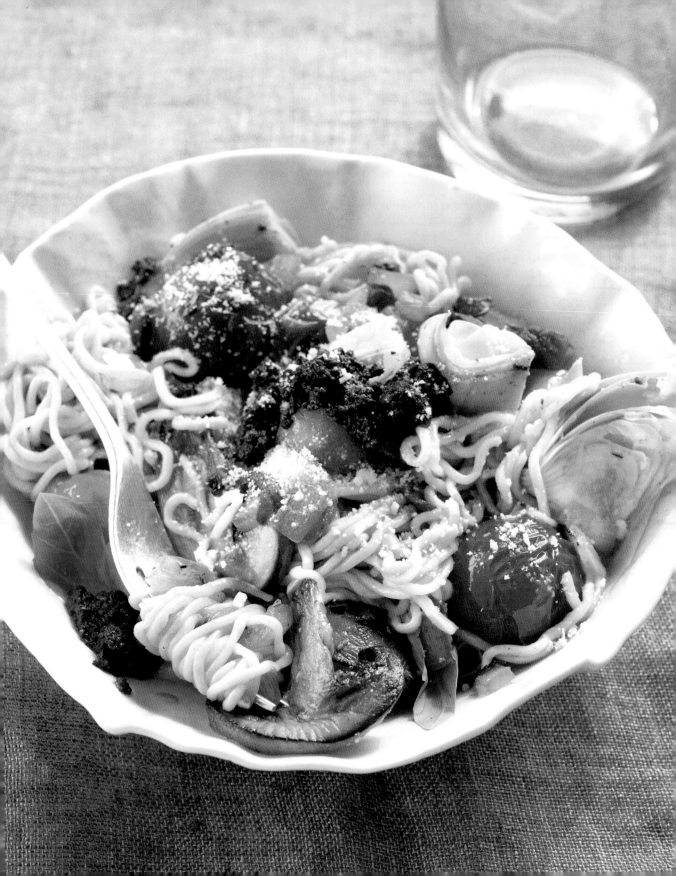

Bow Ties with Garlic and Pesto

■ PREP TIME: 10 MINUTES ■ TOTAL TIME: 25 MINUTES ■ MAKES 4 SERVINGS ■ MUFA: PESTO

You can use any gluten-free small-shaped pasta you like. Elbows or shell macaroni are both good choices.

8 ounces gluten-free brown rice bow tie pasta	¼ cup Pesto (page 84) or store-bought gluten-free pesto
1 tablespoon extra-virgin olive oil	¼ teaspoon salt
1 onion, thinly sliced	8 teaspoons grated Romano cheese
5 cloves garlic, thinly sliced	

1. Bring a large pot of water to a boil over high heat. Cook the pasta according to package directions. Drain.

2. In a large nonstick skillet over medium-high heat, warm the oil. Cook the onion, stirring occasionally, for 5 minutes, or until soft. Stir in the garlic and cook, stirring often, for 2 minutes, or until fragrant. Remove from the heat. Stir in the pasta, pesto, and salt and toss to coat well.

3. Divide the pasta mixture among 4 plates and sprinkle each with 2 teaspoons of the cheese.

Nutrition per serving: 356 calories, 9 g protein, 48 g carbohydrates, 14 g total fat, 4 g saturated fat, 3 g fiber, 357 mg sodium

Make It a FLAT BELLY DIET MEAL

Serve with 2 ounces light tuna packed in water (66).
TOTAL MEAL: 422 calories

Summer Squash Sauté

■ PREP TIME: 10 MINUTES ■ TOTAL TIME: 55 MINUTES ■ MAKES 8 SERVINGS
■ MUFA: SUNFLOWER SEEDS

You can tweak this delicious sauté with whatever seasonal vegetables are available. Onions, peppers, and mushrooms make great toss-ins when you have less squash to work with.

2 tablespoons extra-virgin olive oil
6 cloves garlic, sliced
1 teaspoon red-pepper flakes
3 pounds assorted summer squash (zucchini, yellow squash, etc.), thinly sliced

½ teaspoon salt
1 cup sunflower seeds

1. In a large nonstick skillet set over medium heat, combine the oil, garlic, and red-pepper flakes. Cook, stirring occasionally, for 2 to 3 minutes or until the garlic begins to turn golden. Add the squash and salt. Toss to coat. Cover, reduce the heat to medium-low, and cook for 30 minutes, stirring occasionally, or until the squash begins to break apart.

2. Uncover the pan, increase the heat to medium, and cook for 10 to 12 minutes, or until the liquid is almost gone. Divide evenly among 8 plates and sprinkle with the sunflower seeds.

Nutrition per serving: 63 calories, 2 g protein, 6 g carbohydrates, 4 g total fat, 0.5 g saturated fat, 2 g fiber, 156 mg sodium

Make It a FLAT BELLY DIET MEAL

Serve with Olive-Stuffed Beef Rolls (page 200) (319).
TOTAL MEAL: 382 calories

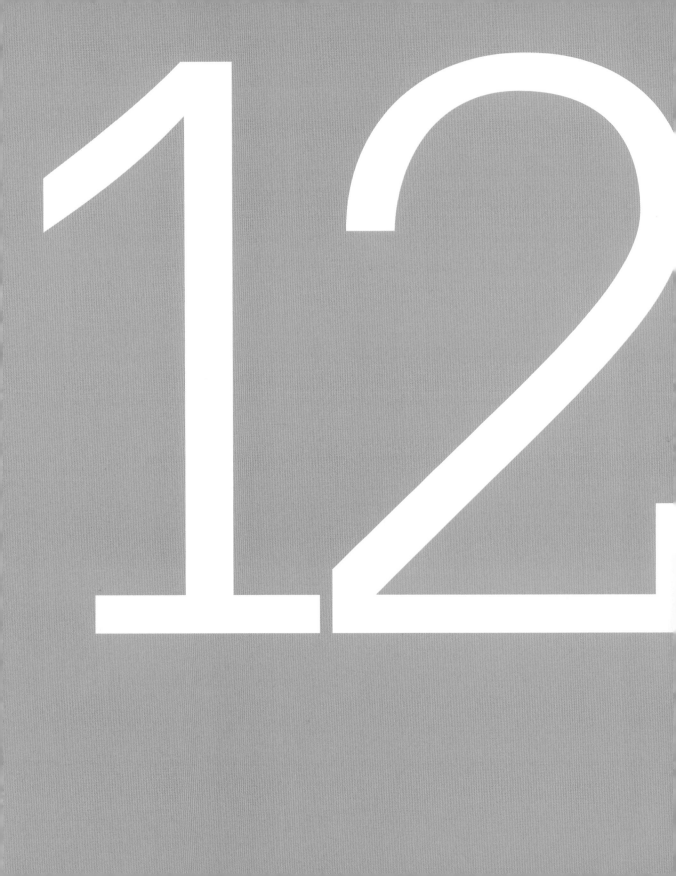

SNACKS

Cumin-Scented Kale Chips

■ PREP TIME: 10 MINUTES ■ TOTAL TIME: 35 MINUTES ■ MAKES 4 SERVINGS ■ MUFA: OLIVE OIL

This healthy, vitamin-packed snack is sure to please even the most finicky eaters. Store the kale chips in an airtight container at room temperature for up to 2 days.

2 bunches kale, tough stems removed and torn into 2" pieces

¼ cup olive oil

¾ teaspoon ground cumin

½ teaspoon coarse salt

1. Preheat the oven to 350°F. Line 2 large baking sheets with parchment paper.

2. In a large bowl, toss the kale with the oil until well coated. Sprinkle with the cumin and salt and mix well. Spread the kale in one layer on the baking sheets. Bake for 20 to 25 minutes, or until crisp.

Nutrition per serving: 178 calories, 4 g protein, 12 g carbohydrates, 15 g total fat, 2 g saturated fat, 2 g fiber, 290 mg sodium

Make It a
FLAT
BELLY
DIET
MEAL

Serve with a turkey burger (150), sliced into cubes and wrapped in a 7" gluten-free tortilla (70), and ¼ cup gluten-free tomato sauce (15). **TOTAL MEAL: 413 calories**

Garlic Tostones

▦ PREP TIME: 10 MINUTES ▦ TOTAL TIME: 20 MINUTES ▦ MAKES 2 SERVINGS ▦ MUFA: CANOLA OIL

Plantains are a staple food in Latin America, similar to potatoes, with a neutral flavor. Using a nonstick skillet is key as you can control the amount of fat used, making this recipe for tostones, or fried plantains, considerably lighter than the traditional Puerto Rican snack.

2 tablespoons canola oil, divided	1 clove garlic, chopped
1 unripe (green) plantain, peeled and sliced into 1" pieces	⅛ teaspoon salt

1. In a large nonstick skillet over medium-high heat, warm 1 tablespoon of the oil. Cook the plantain for 5 minutes, turning the pieces as necessary, until they begin to brown. Remove from the heat.

2. Use the flat bottom of a drinking glass to press and flatten the cut side of each piece.

3. Heat the remaining 1 tablespoon oil over medium-high heat with the garlic. Cook the plantain for 5 minutes longer, turning the pieces as necessary, until they are crisped and brown. Sprinkle with the salt.

Nutrition per serving: 235 calories, 1 g protein, 29 g carbohydrates, 14 g total fat, 1 g saturated fat, 2 g fiber, 149 mg sodium

Make It a
FLAT
BELLY
DIET
MEAL
Serve with a half-serving of Fiesta Casserole (page 189), omitting the avocado (168).
TOTAL MEAL: 403 calories

Olive and White Bean Hummus

■ PREP TIME: 15 MINUTES ■ TOTAL TIME: 15 MINUTES ■ MAKES 8 SERVINGS (½ CUP EACH)
■ MUFA: OLIVES, TAHINI

Serve this naturally gluten-free, high-protein snack on cucumber slices topped with a little chopped fresh mint.

1 can (15½–19 ounces) cannellini beans, rinsed and drained	2 tablespoons olive oil
40 kalamata olives, pitted and chopped	2 cloves garlic
½ cup tahini	½ teaspoon ground cumin
¼ cup lemon juice	¼ teaspoon salt

In a food processor, combine the beans, olives, tahini, lemon juice, oil, garlic, cumin, and salt. Pulse until smooth. If the mixture is too thick, add water, 1 tablespoon at a time, until the hummus reaches the desired consistency.

Nutrition per serving: 207 calories, 4 g protein, 11 g carbohydrates, 17 g total fat, 2 g saturated fat, 2 g fiber, 435 mg sodium

Make It a
FLAT BELLY DIET MEAL
Serve with 4 ounces gluten-free corn tortilla chips (140), 1 large carrot cut into sticks (30), and 1 cup grape tomatoes (30).
TOTAL MEAL: 407 calories

Thai Peanut Dip
with Crunchy Bell Peppers

▦ PREP TIME: 10 MINUTES ▦ TOTAL TIME: 10 MINUTES ▦ MAKES 4 SERVINGS
▦ MUFA: PEANUT BUTTER

**If you prefer to make your own peanut butter, simply puree ½ cup peanuts
with the rest of the ingredients in this recipe.**

½ cup creamy natural peanut butter	2 teaspoons lime juice
¼ cup warm water	½ teaspoon sugar
1 tablespoon gluten-free reduced-sodium soy sauce	2 tablespoons chopped fresh cilantro
	2 red bell peppers, cut into strips

In a medium bowl, combine the peanut butter, water, soy sauce, lime juice, and sugar
until smooth. Stir in the cilantro. Serve with the bell pepper strips.

Nutrition per serving: 224 calories, 8 g protein, 11 g carbohydrates, 16 g total fat, 2 g saturated fat,
3 g fiber, 278 mg sodium

**Make It a
FLAT
BELLY
DIET
MEAL**

Serve with 4 ounces steamed shrimp (112) and 1 cup cooked shirataki
noodles (53).
TOTAL MEAL: 389 calories

Texas "Caviar"

■ PREP TIME: 10 MINUTES ■ TOTAL TIME: 20 MINUTES + CHILLING TIME
■ MAKES 4 SERVINGS ■ MUFA: OLIVE OIL

Black-eyed peas are rich in complex carbohydrates, which play an important role in keeping blood sugar levels steady.

¼ cup olive oil

2 tablespoons apple cider vinegar

1 clove garlic, minced

¼ teaspoon salt

1 can (15 ounces) unsalted black-eyed peas, rinsed and drained

1 green bell pepper, chopped

¼ cup roasted red pepper strips, drained

½ small red onion, finely chopped

2 gluten-free brown rice tortillas, each cut into 8 wedges

1. In a large bowl, whisk together the oil, vinegar, garlic, and salt. Stir in the black-eyed peas, bell pepper, red pepper, and onion.

2. Cover and chill for at least 2 hours, or until ready to serve.

3. Preheat the oven to 400°F. Place the tortilla wedges on a large baking sheet and lightly coat them with cooking spray. Bake for 6 to 8 minutes, or until lightly toasted. Serve with the black-eyed pea mixture.

Nutrition per serving: 249 calories, 5 g protein, 24 g carbohydrates, 15 g total fat, 2 g saturated fat, 4 g fiber, 317 mg sodium

Make It a
FLAT
BELLY
DIET
MEAL
Serve with 3 ounces roasted chicken breast (140) and 2 tablespoons gluten-free barbecue sauce (40).
TOTAL MEAL: 429 calories

Walnut-Apricot Scones

■ PREP TIME: 15 MINUTES ■ TOTAL TIME: 45 MINUTES ■ MAKES 8 SERVINGS
■ MUFA: WALNUTS, CANOLA OIL

These scones are best eaten within a day or two. Freeze leftovers in a resealable food storage bag for up to 3 weeks. Reheat the scones in a 350°F oven for 5 to 10 minutes, or until warm.

2 cups gluten-free all-purpose flour blend	¼ cup canola oil
½ cup + 1 teaspoon sugar	1 egg
2 teaspoons baking powder	½ cup finely chopped walnuts
1 teaspoon xanthan gum	¼ cup dried apricots, chopped (about 8 dried apricot halves)
½ teaspoon salt	2 tablespoons fat-free milk
½ cup buttermilk	

1. Preheat the oven to 400°F. Lightly coat a 9" springform pan with cooking spray.

2. In a large bowl, whisk together the flour, ½ cup sugar, baking powder, xanthan gum, and salt. In a medium bowl, whisk together the buttermilk, oil, and egg. Add to the flour mixture along with the walnuts and apricots and stir just until a soft dough forms.

3. Press the dough into the prepared pan. Score the dough with a knife to form 8 triangles. Brush with the milk and sprinkle with 1 teaspoon sugar.

4. Bake for 20 to 25 minutes, or until lightly browned and a wooden pick inserted in the center comes out clean. Cool for 5 minutes in the pan on a rack. Remove to the rack and cool completely.

Nutrition per serving: 288 calories, 4 g protein, 45 g carbohydrates, 13 g total fat, 1 g saturated fat, 2 g fiber, 282 mg sodium

Make It a FLAT BELLY DIET MEAL

Serve with 8 ounces cappuccino made with 1% milk (73) and 1 cup sliced strawberries (47).

TOTAL MEAL: 408 calories

Almond-Coconut Muffins

■ PREP TIME: 10 MINUTES ■ TOTAL TIME: 35 MINUTES ■ MAKES 12 SERVINGS
■ MUFA: ALMOND MEAL

Both almond flour and almond meal are basically ground almonds. Some brands of almond flour have a finer texture because they are made from almonds that are blanched (their skins are removed) first. They can both be used interchangeably with good results.

1½ cups almond flour/meal	¼ teaspoon salt
½ cup unsweetened shredded coconut	¾ cup sugar
¼ cup sorghum flour	½ cup buttermilk
1½ teaspoons baking powder	⅓ cup canola oil
1 teaspoon xanthan gum	2 eggs
	1 teaspoon pure vanilla extract

1. Preheat the oven to 350°F. Line a 12-cup muffin pan with paper liners or coat it with cooking spray.

2. In a large bowl, whisk together the almond flour, shredded coconut, sorghum flour, baking powder, xanthan gum, and salt. In a medium bowl, whisk together the sugar, buttermilk, oil, eggs, and vanilla until smooth. Add to the flour mixture and stir just until blended.

3. Divide the batter among the muffin cups. Bake for 20 minutes, or until a wooden pick inserted in the center of a muffin comes out clean. Cool in the pan on a rack for 5 minutes. Remove to the rack and cool completely.

Nutrition per serving: 238 calories, 5 g protein, 20 g carbohydrates, 17 g total fat, 3.5 g saturated fat, 2 g fiber, 132 mg sodium

Make It a FLAT BELLY DIET MEAL
Serve with 1 cup 1% milk (102) and ½ cup sliced mango (53).
TOTAL MEAL: 393 calories

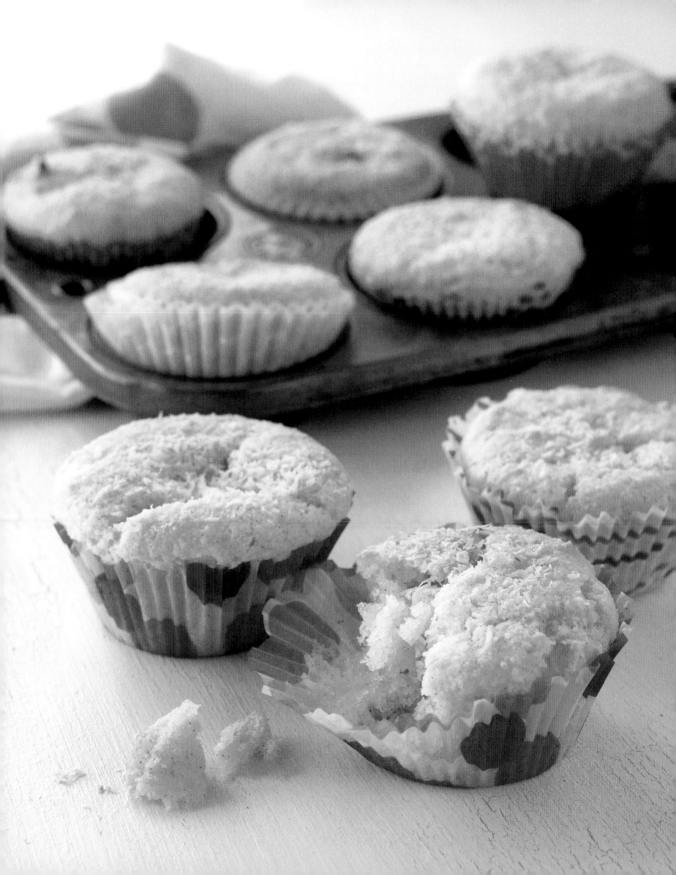

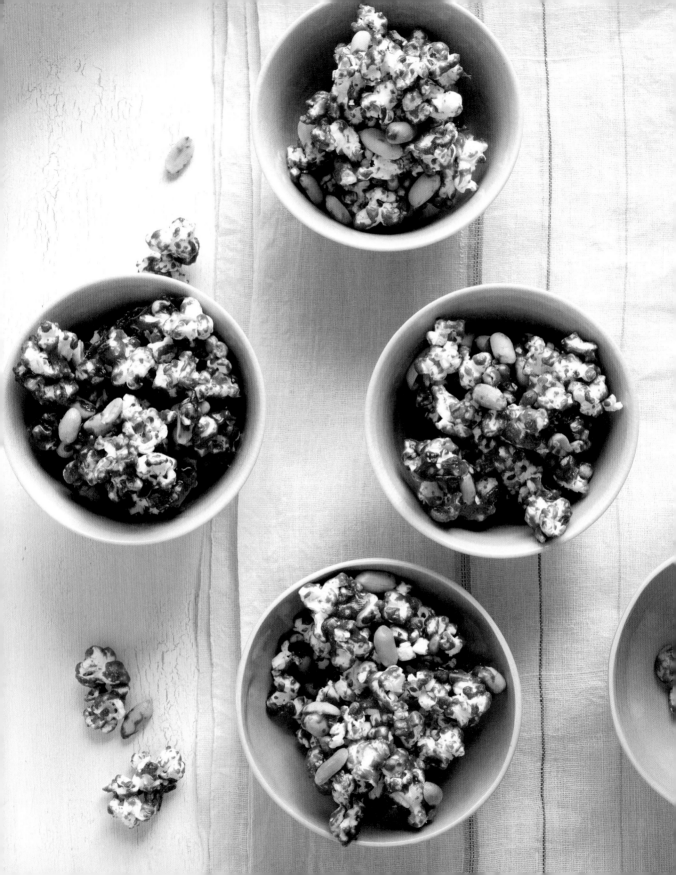

Peanut Caramel Popcorn

■ PREP TIME: 10 MINUTES ■ TOTAL TIME: 1 HOUR ■ MAKES 8 SERVINGS ■ MUFA: PEANUTS

This sweet and crunchy treat is great for movie night in, game day, or packed in pretty tins and given as holiday gifts.

¼ cup packed light brown sugar
¼ cup maple syrup
4 tablespoons butter, softened
1 tablespoon molasses
½ teaspoon salt

2 teaspoons pure vanilla extract
½ teaspoon baking soda
8 cups plain air-popped popcorn
1 cup unsalted dry-roasted peanuts

1. Preheat the oven to 200°F. Coat a large rimmed baking sheet with cooking spray.

2. In a small saucepan, combine the brown sugar, syrup, butter, molasses, and salt. Bring to a boil over high heat. Reduce the heat to medium and cook for 5 minutes, stirring once or twice. Remove from the heat. Stir in the vanilla and baking soda until blended.

3. In a large bowl, combine the popcorn and peanuts. Pour the sugar mixture over, stirring, until well coated. Spread the popcorn mixture evenly onto the baking sheet.

4. Bake, stirring occasionally, for 45 minutes. Cool completely in the pan on a rack. Store the popcorn mixture in an airtight container at room temperature for up to 1 week.

Nutrition per serving: 251 calories, 5 g protein, 26 g carbohydrates, 15 g total fat, 5 g saturated fat, 3 g fiber, 270 mg sodium

Make It a FLAT BELLY DIET MEAL

Serve with a Creamy Mango Frappé (page 285), omitting the flaxseed oil (159).
TOTAL MEAL: 410 calories

Berry-Avocado Smoothie

PREP TIME: 10 MINUTES ■ TOTAL TIME: 10 MINUTES ■ MAKES 2 SERVINGS (1 CUP EACH)
■ MUFA: AVOCADO

For a dairy-free version, use unsweetened almond or coconut milk.

1 cup fresh or frozen blueberries

¾ cup 1% milk

½ cup gluten-free low-fat vanilla frozen yogurt, softened slightly

½ Hass avocado, peeled, pitted, and cubed

1 tablespoon grated lime peel

3 ice cubes

In a blender, combine the blueberries, milk, yogurt, avocado, lime peel, and ice cubes. Puree for about 30 seconds, or until smooth. Pour into 2 tall glasses and serve.

Nutrition per serving: 207 calories, 6 g protein, 30 g carbohydrates, 9 g total fat, 1.5 g saturated fat, 6 g fiber, 76 mg sodium

Make It a FLAT BELLY DIET MEAL
Serve with 1 medium pear, sliced (103), and 1 piece reduced-fat mozzarella string cheese (70).
TOTAL MEAL: 380 calories

Cashew-Ginger Granola

■ PREP TIME: 10 MINUTES ■ TOTAL TIME: 45 MINUTES ■ MAKES 24 SERVINGS ■ MUFA: CASHEWS

Store the granola in the refrigerator in an airtight container for up to 1 month.

3 cups gluten-free rolled oats
2 cups cashews, coarsely chopped
½ cup sunflower seeds
½ cup shelled pumpkin seeds
½ cup packed light brown sugar
⅓ cup maple syrup

¼ cup canola oil
1 tablespoon ground cinnamon
1 tablespoon ground ginger
1 tablespoon pure vanilla extract

1. Preheat the oven to 325°F. Coat a large rimmed baking sheet with cooking spray. Combine the oats, cashews, sunflower seeds, and pumpkin seeds in the pan.

2. In a small saucepan, heat the sugar, maple syrup, oil, cinnamon, and ginger over medium-low heat. Cook, stirring, for 3 minutes, or until the sugar is completely dissolved. Stir in the vanilla. Drizzle over the oat mixture, stirring with a wooden spoon until evenly coated. Spread the mixture evenly out on the pan.

3. Bake, stirring occasionally, for 30 minutes, or until golden brown. Let cool completely.

Nutrition per serving: 181 calories, 5 g protein, 19 g carbohydrates, 10 g total fat, 1.5 g saturated fat, 2 g fiber, 4 mg sodium

Make It a
FLAT
BELLY
DIET
MEAL

Serve in a bowl with 1 cup 1% milk (102) and a medium banana, sliced (105).
TOTAL MEAL: 388 calories

Spice-Roasted Almonds

PREP TIME: 10 MINUTES ▪ TOTAL TIME: 40 MINUTES ▪ MAKES 8 SERVINGS ▪ MUFA: ALMONDS

These spicy, slow-roasted almonds are perfect as an afternoon snack or part of a tapas-style buffet.

1 cup whole blanched almonds	1 teaspoon smoked paprika
2 teaspoons olive oil	1/2 teaspoon ground cumin
1 1/2 teaspoons chopped fresh rosemary	1/4 teaspoon coarse salt

1. Preheat the oven to 300°F.

2. In a small bowl, combine the almonds, oil, rosemary, paprika, cumin, and salt until well mixed.

3. Spread the almond mixture evenly onto a small rimmed baking sheet. Bake, stirring occasionally, for 25 to 30 minutes, or until the almonds are lightly browned. Transfer the pan to a wire rack to cool completely. Store in an airtight container for up to 2 weeks.

Nutrition per serving: 117 calories, 4 g protein, 4 g carbohydrates, 10 g total fat, 1 g saturated fat, 2 g fiber, 65 mg sodium

Make It a FLAT BELLY DIET MEAL

Serve with 1 cup red or green grapes (104), 4 gluten-free multiseed crackers (35), and 2 pieces reduced-fat mozzarella string cheese (140). **TOTAL MEAL: 396 calories**

Curried Cashews

PREP TIME: 5 MINUTES ▪ TOTAL TIME: 10 MINUTES ▪ MAKES 8 SERVINGS ▪ MUFA: CASHEWS

Feel free to substitute pecans or walnuts, if you prefer.

2 teaspoons canola oil

1 cup unsalted dry-roasted cashews

2 teaspoons curry powder

¼ teaspoon salt

Pinch of ground red pepper

In a medium skillet over medium heat, warm the oil. Add the cashews, curry powder, salt, and red pepper. Cook, stirring frequently, for 2 to 3 minutes, or until golden. Serve warm or at room temperature.

Nutrition per serving: 110 calories, 3 g protein, 6 g carbohydrates, 9 g total fat, 1.5 g saturated fat, 1 g fiber, 76 mg sodium

Make It a FLAT BELLY DIET MEAL

Serve with Curried Chicken Waldorf Salad (page 148), omitting the walnuts (313).
TOTAL MEAL: 423 calories

Caramelized Onion and Olive Focaccia

PREP TIME: 25 MINUTES ■ TOTAL TIME: 1 HOUR 15 MINUTES ■ MAKES 8 SERVINGS
■ MUFA: OLIVE OIL, OLIVES

This focaccia is not only great for snacking, but also makes outstanding sandwich bread.

6 tablespoons olive oil, divided

1 large Vidalia onion, chopped

20 kalamata olives, pitted and coarsely chopped

1 tablespoon chopped fresh rosemary

1½ cups gluten-free all-purpose flour blend

2 teaspoons xanthan gum

2 teaspoons sugar

1 envelope (¼ ounce) rapid-rise yeast

½ teaspoon salt

⅔ cup warm water (120°–125°F)

1 egg

1 teaspoon cider vinegar

1. In a medium nonstick skillet over medium-high heat, warm 2 tablespoons of the oil. Cook the onion and olives, stirring occasionally, for 6 to 8 minutes, or until the onions are softened. Remove from the heat. Stir in the rosemary. Let cool.

2. Preheat the oven to 425°F. Coat a 9" springform pan with cooking spray.

3. In a food processor, combine the flour, xanthan gum, sugar, yeast, and salt. Pulse to mix. With the machine running, add the water, egg, vinegar, and 3 tablespoons of the oil. Process for 1 minute, or until the mixture begins to come together.

4. Scrape the dough into the prepared pan and, with oiled hands, press the dough evenly in the pan. Drizzle with the remaining 1 tablespoon oil. Cover loosely with plastic wrap and let rest for 20 minutes. Sprinkle the onion mixture evenly over the top. Bake the focaccia for 15 to 20 minutes, or until the bottom is crusty and the topping is lightly browned. Cut into 8 wedges. Serve warm or at room temperature.

Nutrition per serving: 192 calories, 4 g protein, 23 g carbohydrates, 11 g total fat, 1.5 g saturated fat, 4 g fiber, 313 mg sodium

Make It a FLAT BELLY DIET MEAL Serve with Roast Beef Onion Soup (page 98) (205).
TOTAL MEAL: 397 calories

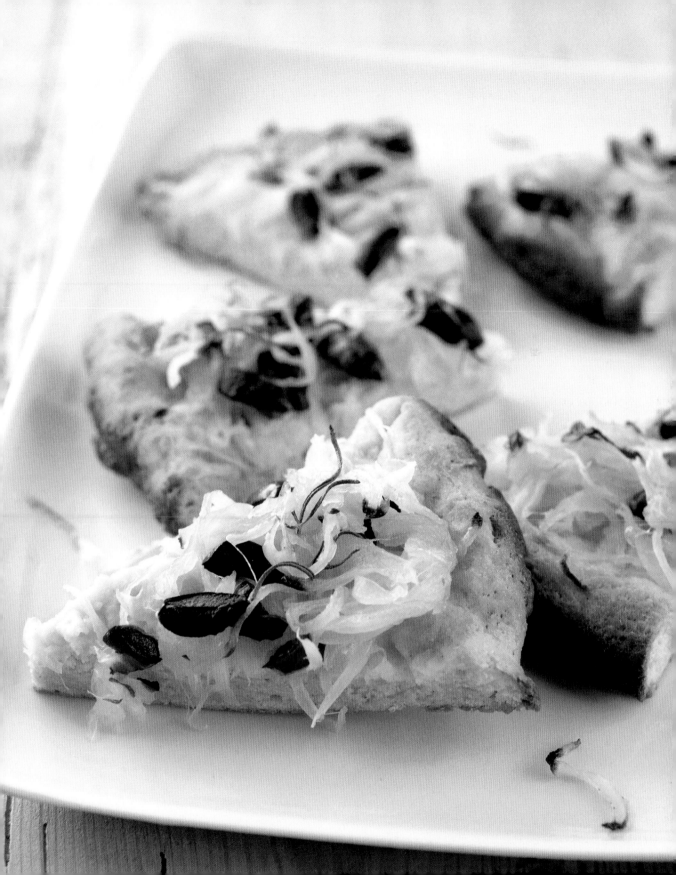

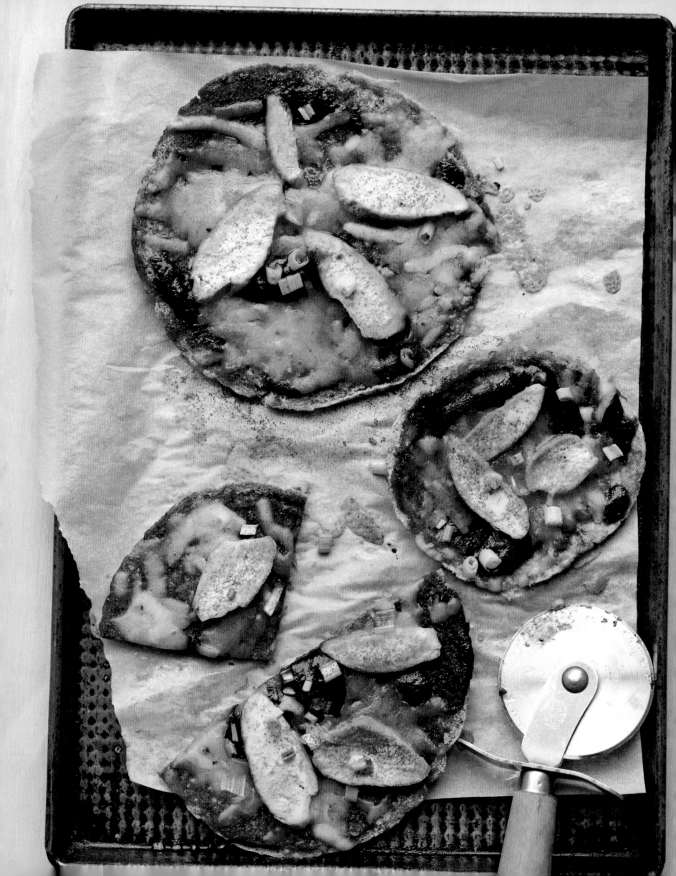

Barbecue Chicken Pizzas

PREP TIME: 10 MINUTES ▦ TOTAL TIME: 20 MINUTES ▦ MAKES 2 SERVINGS ▦ MUFA: OLIVE OIL

When you need a quick pizza fix, this recipe will do the trick, especially if you love thin crusts.

- 2 gluten-free tortillas (8" diameter)
- 2 tablespoons olive oil
- 2 tablespoons gluten-free barbecue sauce
- ¼ cup shredded reduced-fat pepper Jack cheese
- 4 ounces cooked thinly sliced chicken breast
- 2 scallions, thinly sliced

1. Preheat the oven to 400°F.

2. Place the tortillas on a baking sheet. Brush each tortilla with 1 tablespoon of the oil. Top each with half of the barbecue sauce, cheese, chicken, and onion.

3. Bake for 7 minutes, or until the toppings are hot and the cheese is melted. To serve, cut each pizza into 4 wedges.

Nutrition per serving: 357 calories, 21 g protein, 25 g carbohydrates, 20 g total fat, 3.5 g saturated fat, 6 g fiber, 383 mg sodium

Make It a
FLAT
BELLY
DIET
MEAL

Serve with a salad made from ½ cucumber, sliced (12), tossed with 1 cup grape tomatoes (30) and 2 tablespoons minced red onion (12).
TOTAL MEAL: 411 calories

13

DESSERTS

Almond-Berry Crisp

▨ PREP TIME: 10 MINUTES ▨ TOTAL TIME: 30 MINUTES ▨ MAKES 4 SERVINGS ▨ MUFA: ALMOND MEAL

Any mixture of seasonal fruits works well. Chopped plums or peaches would be just as delicious.

1 cup almond meal

3 tablespoons packed brown sugar

2 tablespoons gluten-free
tapioca flour

2 tablespoons softened butter

1 teaspoon ground cinnamon

2 cups blueberries

1 cup raspberries

1 cup blackberries

1. Preheat the oven to 400°F. Coat a 1½-quart baking dish with cooking spray.

2. In a small bowl, combine the almond meal, brown sugar, flour, butter, and cinnamon until coarse crumbs form.

3. Place the berries in the bottom of the baking dish. Sprinkle the almond mixture evenly over the berries.

4. Bake for 20 minutes, or until the filling is hot and the topping is browned and bubbly.

Nutrition per serving: 337 calories, 7 g protein, 38 g carbohydrates, 20 g total fat, 5 g saturated fat, 9 g fiber, 5 mg sodium

Make It a
FLAT
BELLY
DIET
MEAL

Serve with 1 cup fat-free milk (83).

TOTAL MEAL: 420 calories

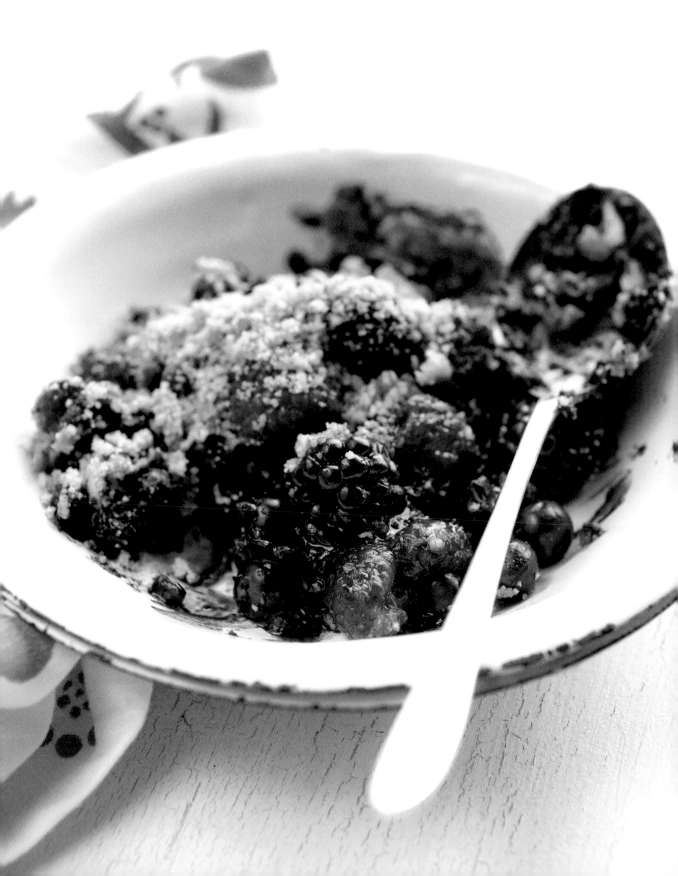

Roast Peaches with Pistachio-Streusel Topping

▦ PREP TIME: 10 MINUTES ▦ TOTAL TIME: 40 MINUTES ▦ MAKES 4 SERVINGS ▦ MUFA: PISTACHIOS

Roasting peaches enhances their sweetness, and the streusel topping adds a nutty crunch.

4 peaches, halved and pitted

3 tablespoons butter, at room temperature

2 tablespoons packed dark brown sugar

$\frac{1}{2}$ teaspoon ground cinnamon

$\frac{1}{2}$ cup unsalted pistachios, finely chopped

1. Preheat the oven to 375°F. Coat a 13" x 9" baking dish with cooking spray. Place the peach halves, cut side up, in the dish.

2. In a medium bowl, combine the butter, brown sugar, and cinnamon until blended. Stir in the pistachios. Rub the mixture together with your fingers until it resembles coarse crumbs.

3. Sprinkle the crumb mixture evenly over the peaches. Bake for 25 to 30 minutes, or until the peaches are tender and the top is lightly golden.

Nutrition per serving: 251 calories, 4 g protein, 26 g carbohydrates, 16 g total fat, 6 g saturated fat, 4 g fiber, 65 mg sodium

Make It a FLAT BELLY DIET MEAL } Serve with 6 ounces fat-free vanilla yogurt (155). **TOTAL MEAL: 406 calories**

Peach and Raspberry Tart with Almond Crust

■ PREP TIME: 15 MINUTES ■ TOTAL TIME: 1 HOUR 45 MINUTES ■ MAKES 8 SERVINGS
■ MUFA: ALMOND FLOUR

After placing the dough in the pan, prevent it from sticking to your hands by placing a piece of plastic wrap over the dough and pressing it evenly into the pan. Remove and discard the plastic wrap before filling.

2 cups blanched almond flour	2 tablespoons cold water
2 teaspoons grated lemon peel	¾ cup peach fruit spread
⅛ teaspoon salt	1½ tablespoons cornstarch
1 egg white, lightly beaten	1½ pounds firm ripe peaches, sliced
2 tablespoons canola oil	¾ cup fresh raspberries

1. In a food processor, combine the flour, lemon peel, and salt. Pulse to mix. With the machine running, add the egg white, oil, and water, and pulse until a soft dough forms. Gather the mixture into a ball and press into a thick disk. Transfer the dough to a 9" tart pan with a removable bottom. Firmly press the dough against the bottom and up the sides of the pan. Cover loosely with plastic wrap and refrigerate for 15 minutes.

2. Preheat the oven to 375°F.

3. In a large bowl, combine the fruit spread and cornstarch until blended. Add the peaches and raspberries and toss gently to mix. Spoon into the prepared crust. Bake for 1 hour 15 minutes, or until the juices are bubbling. Cool completely on a rack.

Nutrition per serving: 300 calories, 7 g protein, 33 g carbohydrates, 18 g total fat, 1 g saturated fat, 6 g fiber, 54 mg sodium

Make It a
FLAT
BELLY
DIET
MEAL

Serve with 8 ounces cappuccino made with 1% milk (73).
TOTAL MEAL: 373 calories

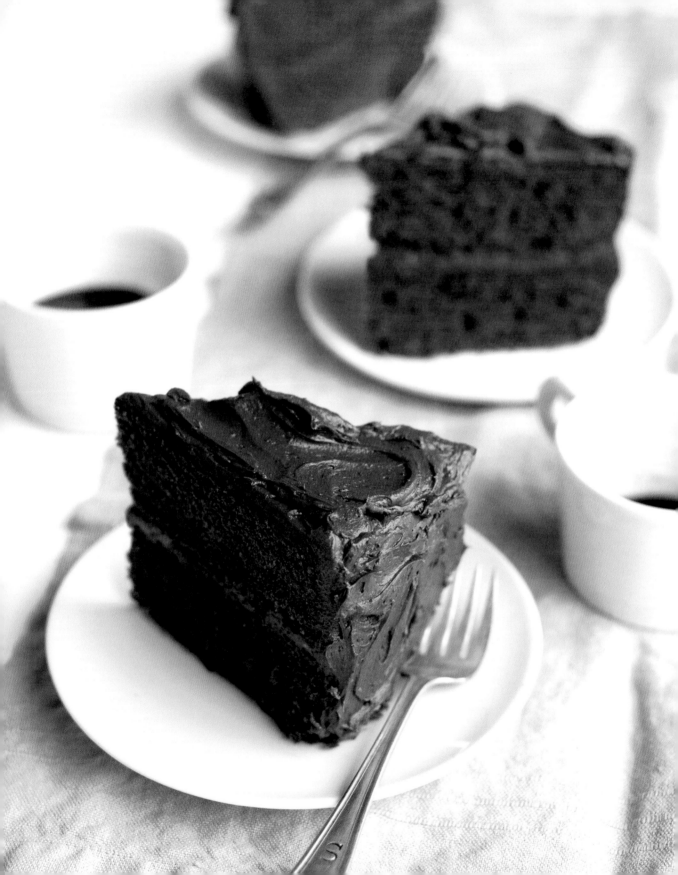

Mocha Chocolate Cake

■ PREP TIME: 10 MINUTES ■ TOTAL TIME: 50 MINUTES + COOLING TIME
■ MAKES 16 SERVINGS ■ MUFA: CANOLA OIL

Various gluten-free flour blends yield different results, so experiment to find your favorite.

CAKE

- 3 cups gluten-free all-purpose flour blend
- 1½ cups granulated sugar
- 1 tablespoon baking soda
- 1 teaspoon xanthan gum
- 1 teaspoon salt
- 1 cup unsweetened cocoa powder, sifted
- 1 cup canola oil
- 1½ cups buttermilk
- 2 eggs
- 1½ cups freshly brewed decaffeinated coffee
- 1 tablespoon pure vanilla extract

CHOCOLATE BUTTERCREAM FROSTING

- ½ cup butter, softened
- ½ cup fat-free cream cheese, softened
- 1 cup confectioners' sugar, sifted
- ½ cup unsweetened cocoa powder, sifted
- 1 teaspoon pure vanilla extract

1. Preheat the oven to 350°F. Coat two 9" round cake pans with cooking spray.

2. **To make the cake:** In a large bowl, mix together the flour, granulated sugar, baking soda, xanthan gum, salt, and cocoa powder with an electric mixer at medium speed until well blended. With the mixer on low speed, beat in the oil and buttermilk until just combined. Beat in the eggs, one at a time, until blended. Add the coffee and vanilla and beat just until blended.

3. Spread the batter into the prepared pans. Bake for 40 minutes, or until a wooden pick inserted in the center comes out clean. Place the pans on a rack and let cool completely, about 1 hour.

4. **To make the frosting:** Meanwhile, in a large bowl and with clean beaters, beat the butter and cream cheese until smooth. Add the confectioners' sugar and cocoa powder, and beat until thoroughly blended (it will look dry and clumpy). Add the vanilla and beat until blended, smooth, and glossy.

(continued)

5. Place 1 cooled cake layer on a serving plate. Evenly spread the top with frosting. Top with the remaining cake layer and spread the top with frosting. Spread the remaining frosting over the sides.

Nutrition per serving: 402 calories, 5 g protein, 50 g carbohydrates, 23 g total fat, 6 g saturated fat, 7 g fiber, 512 mg sodium

Make It a
FLAT
BELLY   A single serving of this recipe counts as a Flat Belly Diet Meal without
DIET   any add-ons!
MEAL

Olive Oil Cornmeal Cake

■ PREP TIME: 10 MINUTES ■ TOTAL TIME: 40 MINUTES + COOLING TIME
■ MAKES 12 SERVINGS ■ MUFA: ALMOND MEAL

This cake is moist and delicious, with just a hint of orange. If you'd like the flavor a little more pronounced, add ½ teaspoon pure gluten-free orange extract to the batter.

1½ cups almond meal	½ cup buttermilk
½ cup gluten-free yellow cornmeal	⅓ cup olive oil
1½ teaspoons baking powder	2 large eggs
½ teaspoon salt	1 tablespoon grated orange peel
¾ cup sugar	

1. Preheat the oven to 350°F. Coat a 9" springform pan with cooking spray.

2. In a medium bowl, combine the almond meal, cornmeal, baking powder, and salt. In a large bowl, whisk together the sugar, buttermilk, oil, eggs, and orange peel. Stir into the almond mixture until just combined.

3. Pour the batter into the prepared pan. Bake for 25 to 30 minutes, or until a wooden pick inserted in the center comes out with a few moist crumbs attached. Cool for 10 minutes in the pan on a rack. Remove to the rack and cool completely.

Nutrition per serving: 224 calories, 5 g protein, 22 g carbohydrates, 14 g total fat, 2 g saturated fat, 2 g fiber, 193 mg sodium

Make It a FLAT BELLY DIET MEAL   Serve with ½ cup fresh pineapple chunks (41) and 2 tablespoons semisweet chocolate chips, melted and drizzled over the cake (104). **TOTAL MEAL: 369 calories**

Banana and Dark Chocolate Chip Cupcakes

■ PREP TIME: 15 MINUTES ■ TOTAL TIME: 40 MINUTES ■ MAKES 12 SERVINGS ■ MUFA: WALNUTS

If you prefer to make this a quick bread, bake in an 8" x 4" loaf pan for 35 to 40 minutes, or until a wooden pick inserted in the center comes out clean.

1 cup millet flour	¾ cup sugar
¼ cup brown rice flour	⅓ cup canola oil
¼ cup sorghum flour	2 large eggs
1½ teaspoons baking powder	1 teaspoon pure vanilla extract
1 teaspoon xanthan gum	¾ cup walnuts, finely chopped
¼ teaspoon salt	½ cup dark chocolate chips
2 ripe medium bananas, mashed	

1. Preheat the oven to 350°F. Line a 12-cup muffin pan with paper liners or coat it with cooking spray.

2. In a large bowl, whisk together the millet, brown rice flour, sorghum flour, baking powder, xanthan gum, and salt. In a medium bowl, combine the bananas, sugar, oil, eggs, and vanilla until smooth. Add to the flour mixture and stir just until blended. Stir in the nuts and chocolate chips.

3. Divide the batter among the prepared muffin cups. Bake for 20 to 25 minutes, or until a wooden pick inserted in the center of a muffin comes out clean. Cool in the pan on a rack for 5 minutes. Remove to the rack and cool completely.

Nutrition per serving: 285 calories, 5 g protein, 35 g carbohydrates, 16 g total fat, 3 g saturated fat, 3 g fiber, 130 mg sodium

Make It a FLAT BELLY DIET MEAL

Serve with 1 cup sliced mango (107).
TOTAL MEAL: 392 calories

No-Bake Almond Butter Bars

■ PREP TIME: 10 MINUTES ■ TOTAL TIME: 35 MINUTES + COOLING TIME
■ MAKES 6 SERVINGS ■ MUFA: ALMONDS, ALMOND BUTTER, CHOCOLATE CHIPS

Think of these treats as a cross between two childhood classics—s'mores and Rice Krispies Treats. Unlike those favorites, however, these are made with gluten-free whole grain cereal. Store in an airtight container at room temperature for up to 3 days.

1 tablespoon butter	3 cups gluten-free rice squares cereal
20 standard-size gluten-free marshmallows	½ cup sliced almonds, chopped
2 tablespoons almond butter	¼ cup semisweet chocolate chips

1. Coat an 8″ x 8″ baking pan with cooking spray.

2. In a large nonstick saucepan, melt the butter over medium heat. Add the marshmallows and cook, stirring, for 4 to 5 minutes, or until melted. Stir in the almond butter, stirring until well combined and smooth. Remove the saucepan from the heat, add the cereal and chopped almonds, and stir until well coated.

3. Transfer to the prepared pan, using a rubber spatula if needed. Place a piece of waxed paper coated with cooking spray over the top and press down with your hand to flatten. Cool for 20 minutes.

4. Remove the cereal square from the pan and set on a rack over a sheet of waxed paper. Place the chocolate chips in a small microwaveable bowl and microwave in 5-second increments, stirring, for 20 to 25 seconds, or until melted. Using a small spoon, drizzle the chocolate in a zig-zag pattern over the cereal square. Cool completely for 30 to 35 minutes, or until the chocolate is set. Cut into 6 bars.

Nutrition per serving: 239 calories, 4 g protein, 34 g carbohydrates, 11 g total fat, 3 g saturated fat, 2 g fiber, 178 mg sodium

Make It a
FLAT
BELLY
DIET
MEAL
Serve with ½ cup fat-free ricotta cheese (100) drizzled with 1 teaspoon honey (21) and ½ cup blackberries (31).
TOTAL MEAL: 391 calories

Cashew Brownies

■ PREP TIME: 10 MINUTES ■ TOTAL TIME: 30 MINUTES + COOLING TIME
■ MAKES 8 SERVINGS ■ MUFA: CASHEWS

These brownies are delicious all by themselves, or with a scoop of reduced-fat vanilla frozen yogurt and a drizzle of caramel sauce.

½ cup gluten-free all-purpose flour blend

⅓ cup unsweetened cocoa powder

½ teaspoon baking powder

½ teaspoon xanthan gum

¼ teaspoon salt

½ cup sugar

¼ cup canola oil

¼ cup warm water

1 large egg

1 egg white

1 teaspoon pure vanilla extract

1 cup cashews, chopped

¼ cup semisweet chocolate chips

1. Preheat the oven to 350°F. Coat an 8″ x 8″ baking pan with cooking spray.

2. In a medium bowl, combine the flour, cocoa powder, baking powder, xanthan gum, and salt. In a small bowl, whisk together the sugar, oil, water, egg, egg white, and vanilla until smooth. Pour into the flour mixture and stir until just blended. Stir in the cashews and chocolate chips.

3. Evenly spread the batter into the prepared pan. Bake for 20 minutes, or until a wooden pick inserted near the edge comes out with a few moist crumbs attached. Cool in the pan for 15 minutes. Transfer to a rack and let cool completely. Cut into 8 squares.

Nutrition per serving: 290 calories, 5 g protein, 32 g carbohydrates, 18 g total fat, 4 g saturated fat, 3 g fiber, 127 mg sodium

Make It a
FLAT
BELLY
DIET
MEAL
} Serve with 1 cup pitted sweet cherries (90).
TOTAL MEAL: 380 calories

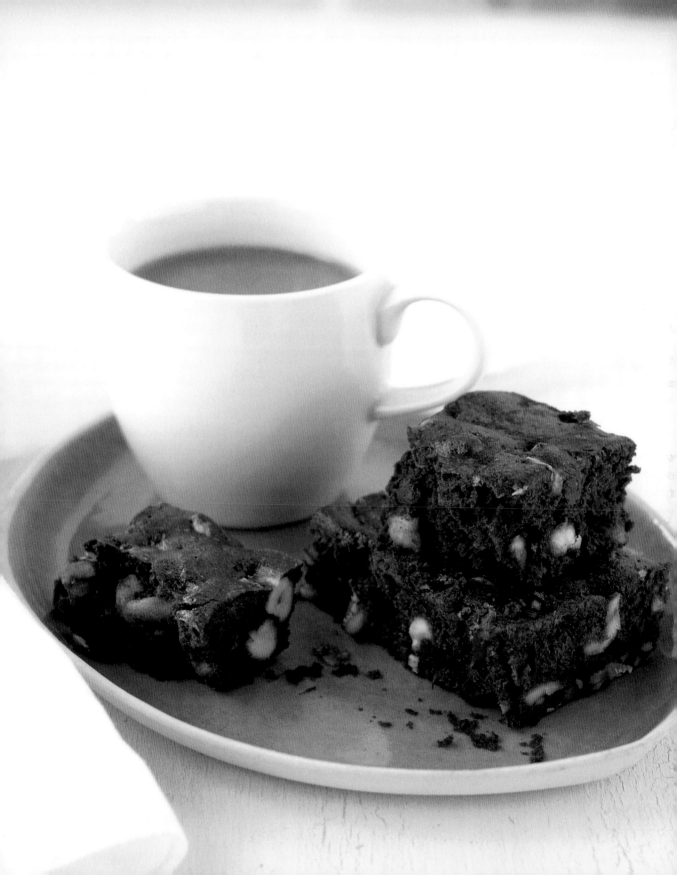

Dried Fruit and Almond Drops

■ PREP TIME: 10 MINUTES ■ TOTAL TIME: 1 HOUR 35 MINUTES + CHILLING TIME
■ MAKES 6 SERVINGS ■ MUFA: ALMONDS

Use any combination of dried fruit you like, such as pitted dates or dried figs—or even try dried papaya or mango bits.

1¼ cups sugar

¼ cup water

1 cup dried mixed fruit, finely chopped

1 tablespoon grated orange peel

¼ teaspoon pure almond extract

¾ cup whole blanched almonds, finely chopped, divided

1. In a small saucepan, bring the sugar and water to a boil over medium-high heat. Cook, stirring occasionally, for 5 to 6 minutes, or until the sugar melts and the syrup is thick enough to coat the back of a spoon.

2. Remove from the heat and stir in the dried fruit, orange peel, and almond extract. Let stand for 20 minutes, or until still warm but not hot. Add ¼ cup of the almonds and stir until combined. Chill for 1 hour.

3. Divide the mixture into 30 equal portions and roll each into a small ball. Place the remaining ½ cup almonds in a bowl and roll each ball in the nuts to coat. Cover and chill for 2 hours to allow to set.

Nutrition per serving: 336 calories, 5 g protein, 63 g carbohydrates, 9 g total fat, 1 g saturated fat, 4 g fiber, 46 mg sodium

Make It a
FLAT
BELLY
DIET
MEAL

Serve with 8 ounces cappuccino made with 1% milk (73).
TOTAL MEAL: 409 calories

Peanut Butter–Chocolate Chunk Cookies

■ PREP TIME: 15 MINUTES ■ TOTAL TIME: 35 MINUTES ■ MAKES 8 SERVINGS
■ MUFA: PEANUT BUTTER

This recipe makes 8 large cookies. If you prefer smaller cookies, drop the dough by heaping tablespoons onto the baking sheet, flatten them slightly, and bake for 12 to 15 minutes, or until set.

1 cup creamy natural peanut butter	1 teaspoon baking soda
½ cup + 3 tablespoons sugar	½ cup chopped semisweet chocolate chunks
1 egg white	
1 teaspoon pure vanilla extract	½ cup unsalted dry-roasted peanuts, chopped

1. Preheat the oven to 350°F. Line 2 large baking sheets with parchment paper.

2. In a large bowl, combine the peanut butter, ½ cup sugar, the egg white, vanilla, and baking soda until blended. Stir in the chopped chocolate and peanuts.

3. Sprinkle the 3 tablespoons sugar on a small plate. Roll the dough, by scant ¼ cups, into 8 balls. Roll each ball into the sugar and place 3" apart on the baking sheets. Flatten each to a 4" round. With the back of a fork, lightly press down on the rounds in a crisscross pattern.

4. Bake for 20 minutes, or until lightly browned at the edges. Cool on the baking sheets for 5 minutes. Transfer to a rack and cool completely.

Nutrition per serving: 394 calories, 10 g protein, 36 g carbohydrates, 25 g total fat, 5 g saturated fat, 4 g fiber, 128 mg sodium

Make It a
FLAT
BELLY
DIET
MEAL

A single serving of this recipe counts as a Flat Belly Diet Meal without any add-ons!

Coconut-Almond Macaroons

■ PREP TIME: 10 MINUTES ■ TOTAL TIME: 40 MINUTES + COOLING TIME
■ MAKES 6 SERVINGS ■ MUFA: ALMONDS

If you'd like to indulge, once the cookies have cooled, melt ¼ cup semisweet chocolate chips and drizzle them over the cookies.

4 egg whites, at room temperature

1½ cups unsweetened shredded coconut

½ cup sugar

¾ cup sliced almonds, coarsely chopped

½ teaspoon pure vanilla extract

1. Preheat the oven to 325°F. Line a large baking sheet with parchment paper.

2. In a large bowl, whisk the egg whites until soft peaks form. Add the coconut, sugar, almonds, and vanilla until well mixed.

3. Drop the mixture, by rounded tablespoons, onto the prepared sheet about 1" apart, to make a total of 18 cookies. Bake for 25 to 30 minutes, or until lightly browned around the edges. Cool on the baking sheet for 15 minutes, or until the macaroons are firm.

Nutrition per serving: 302 calories, 6 g protein, 25 g carbohydrates, 20 g total fat, 13 g saturated fat, 4 g fiber, 44 mg sodium

Make It a
FLAT
BELLY
DIET
MEAL

Serve with 1 medium apple, sliced (95).
TOTAL MEAL: 397 calories

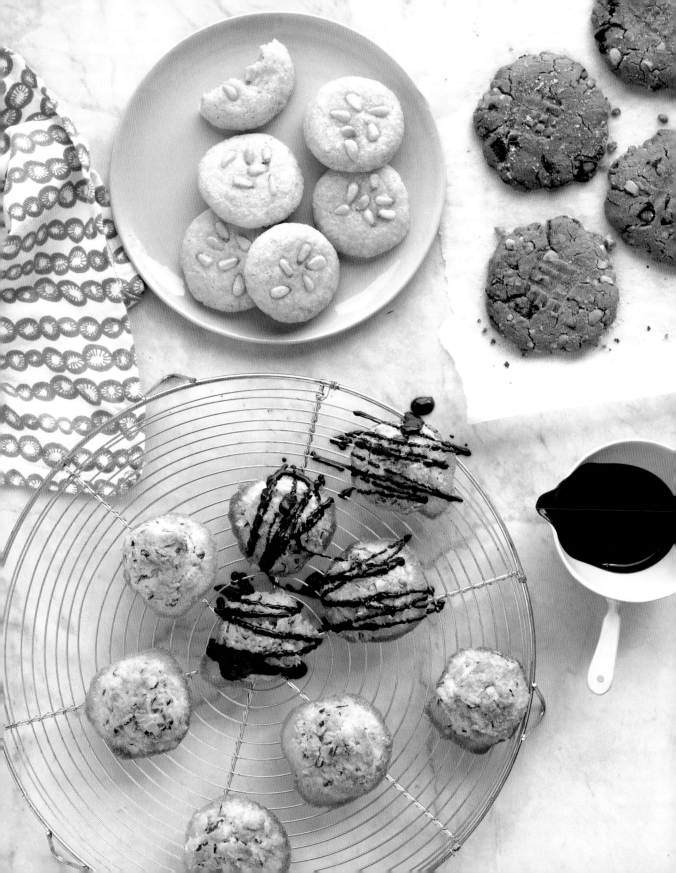

Lemon–Pine Nut Cookies

■ PREP TIME: 10 MINUTES ■ TOTAL TIME: 25 MINUTES ■ MAKES 12 SERVINGS ■ MUFA: PINE NUTS

In Italian, these chewy delights are known as pignoli cookies. If you like a crisper cookie, bake them for 8 to 10 minutes longer.

1 cup almond meal	1 egg white
¾ cup pine nuts, divided	1 tablespoon grated lemon peel
½ cup sugar	Pinch of salt

1. Preheat the oven to 300°F. Line 2 large baking sheets with parchment paper.

2. In a food processor, combine the almond meal, ½ cup of the pine nuts, and the sugar. Pulse for 30 seconds, or until finely ground. Add the egg white, lemon peel, and salt. Pulse until the mixture begins to form a dough.

3. Roll the dough by rounded teaspoons into 24 balls (¾" diameter) and place 1" apart on the baking sheets. Flatten the cookies into 1½" rounds. Sprinkle with the remaining ¼ cup pine nuts and lightly press to make the nuts adhere.

4. Bake for 15 minutes, or until lightly golden. Cool completely on the baking sheets on racks. Carefully peel the cookies off the parchment. Store at room temperature in an airtight container for up to 2 weeks.

Nutrition per serving: 144 calories, 3 g protein, 12 g carbohydrates, 10 g total fat, 1 g saturated fat, 1 g fiber, 20 mg sodium

Make It a
FLAT
BELLY
DIET
MEAL
Serve with 8 ounces cappuccino made with 1% milk (73) and 6 ounces fat-free vanilla yogurt (155) mixed with 1 cup sliced strawberries (47). **TOTAL MEAL: 419 calories**

Walnut Meringues

■ PREP TIME: 10 MINUTES ■ TOTAL TIME: 3 HOURS 10 MINUTES ■ MAKES 6 SERVINGS
■ MUFA: WALNUTS

Don't make these cookies on a humid day. The humidity will prevent them from getting crisp.

4 egg whites, at room temperature
¼ teaspoon cream of tartar
½ cup sugar

1 teaspoon pure vanilla extract
¾ cup ground walnuts

1. Preheat the oven to 200°F. Line 2 large baking sheets with parchment paper.

2. In a large bowl, with an electric mixer on low speed, beat the egg whites and cream of tartar until foamy. Add the sugar, 2 tablespoons at a time, and the vanilla, and beat on high speed for 3 to 4 minutes, or until the whites stand in stiff glossy peaks. With a rubber spatula, fold in the walnuts. Drop the meringues by rounded tablespoons onto the prepared sheets.

3. Bake for 2 hours, or until the meringues are dried and crisp. Turn the oven off and leave them in the oven for 1 hour.

4. Transfer the meringues to racks to cool completely. Carefully peel the meringues off the parchment. Store at room temperature in an airtight container for up to 2 weeks.

Nutrition per serving: 143 calories, 4 g protein, 18 g carbohydrates, 7 g total fat, 1 g saturated fat, 1 g fiber, 37 mg sodium

Make It a FLAT BELLY DIET MEAL } Serve with 1 cup red or green grapes (104), ½ cup fresh pineapple chunks (41), 1 cup fresh blackberries (62), and 1 cup fresh blueberries (84).
TOTAL MEAL: 434 calories

Pecan-Coconut Clusters

PREP TIME: 5 MINUTES ▓ TOTAL TIME: 15 MINUTES ▓ MAKES 8 SERVINGS ▓ MUFA: PECANS

Making these crunchy caramelized candies is easy but does require attention. Make sure there are pot holders and heatproof utensils at hand. And never directly touch the sugar syrup with bare hands.

3 tablespoons sugar

1 tablespoon light corn syrup

1 cup pecans, coarsely chopped

2 tablespoons unsweetened flaked coconut

1. Coat a baking sheet with cooking spray.

2. In a large heavy-bottomed skillet, add the sugar. Drizzle the corn syrup evenly over the sugar and set over medium heat. Cook, without stirring, for 2 to 3 minutes, or until the sugar starts to melt. Tip the pan gently to help submerge any sugar that isn't dissolved. Scatter the nuts and coconut on top. Cook, stirring occasionally with a heatproof rubber spatula, for 6 to 7 minutes, or until the nuts turn a caramel color.

3. Immediately scrape the mixture out onto the baking sheet. Use 2 spatulas to divide it into 16 clusters, pressing the nuts together as you work. Do not touch the mixture while hot. Set aside to cool. Store in an airtight container at room temperature.

Nutrition per serving: 134 calories, 1 g protein, 9 g carbohydrates, 11 g total fat, 2 g saturated fat, 1 g fiber, 2 mg sodium

Make It a
FLAT
BELLY
DIET
MEAL

Serve with 1 cup 1% milk (102) and 1 medium apple (97) drizzled with 2 teaspoons honey (42).
TOTAL MEAL: 375 calories

Sesame-Honey Crunch

▓ PREP TIME: 5 MINUTES ▓ TOTAL TIME: 45 MINUTES ▓ MAKES 12 SERVINGS ▓ MUFA: SESAME SEEDS

Candy making is easy and does not require a lot of equipment. However, a good candy thermometer is a useful tool because time and temperature are critical for good results. Choose one with a metal clamp that attaches to the side of the pan.

1½ cups sesame seeds	1 teaspoon pure vanilla extract
½ cup honey	¼ teaspoon salt
½ cup packed light brown sugar	

1. Line an 8" x 8" baking pan with parchment paper or waxed paper and coat with cooking spray.

2. In a large skillet, toast the sesame seeds over medium heat, stirring often, for 3 minutes or until lightly golden. Transfer to a small bowl and set aside.

3. In a medium heavy-bottomed saucepan, bring the honey and sugar to a boil over medium-high heat. Cook, stirring constantly, for 10 minutes, or until the mixture registers 250°F on a candy thermometer. Stir in the vanilla, salt, and the reserved seeds and cook, stirring often, for 4 minutes, or until the mixture reaches 275°F on the thermometer.

4. Pour into the prepared pan and let stand for 15 to 20 minutes or until still warm but cool enough to handle. Turn the candy out onto a cutting board and cut into 24 pieces. Cool to room temperature.

Nutrition per serving: 182 calories, 3 g protein, 25 g carbohydrates, 9 g total fat, 1 g saturated fat, 2 g fiber, 54 mg sodium

Make It a FLAT BELLY DIET MEAL

Serve with 1 cup 0% Greek yogurt (120) drizzled with 2 teaspoons honey (42) and ½ cup each fresh blueberries (42) and fresh blackberries (31).
TOTAL MEAL: 417 calories

Dark Chocolate Mint Pudding

■ PREP TIME: 10 MINUTES ■ TOTAL TIME: 15 MINUTES + CHILLING TIME
■ MAKES 6 SERVINGS (½ CUP EACH) ■ MUFA: SEMISWEET CHOCOLATE CHIPS

For best results, prepare the pudding a day ahead, then cover and refrigerate overnight to let the flavors meld.

¼ cup sugar

¼ cup unsweetened cocoa powder

2 tablespoons cornstarch

¼ teaspoon salt

3 cups 1% milk

1½ cups semisweet chocolate chips

1½ teaspoons peppermint extract

1. In a medium saucepan, combine the sugar, cocoa powder, cornstarch, and salt. Whisk in the milk and bring to a boil over high heat. Reduce the heat to medium and cook, whisking, for 4 minutes, or until the pudding begins to thicken.

2. Remove from the heat and stir in the chocolate chips and peppermint. Transfer to a bowl. Cover and chill for at least 2 hours, or until set.

Nutrition per serving: 304 calories, 7 g protein, 46 g carbohydrates, 14 g total fat, 9 g saturated fat, 4 g fiber, 156 mg sodium

Make It a
FLAT
BELLY
DIET
MEAL
} Serve with 1½ cups cantaloupe balls (90).
TOTAL MEAL: 394 calories

Dark Chocolate Fudge Pops

■ PREP TIME: 10 MINUTES ■ TOTAL TIME: 15 MINUTES + FREEZING TIME
■ MAKES 8 SERVINGS ■ MUFA: SEMISWEET CHOCOLATE CHIPS

To loosen the ice pops from the mold, dip the mold in warm water for about 10 seconds.

2 cups 1% milk	1½ cups semisweet chocolate chips
¼ cup unsweetened cocoa powder	2 teaspoons pure vanilla extract

1. In a medium saucepan, bring the milk to a simmer over medium-high heat. Add the cocoa powder and cook, whisking often, for 5 minutes, or until the cocoa is completely dissolved.

2. Remove the saucepan from the heat. Add the chocolate chips and vanilla, whisking until smooth. Cool to room temperature.

3. Divide the chocolate mixture among 8 (⅓-cup) ice pop molds. Top with mold covers and freeze until firm, about 6 hours or overnight.

Nutrition per serving: 245 calories, 6 g protein, 32 g carbohydrates, 13 g total fat, 8 g saturated fat, 3 g fiber, 28 mg sodium

Make It a FLAT BELLY DIET MEAL

Serve with ¾ cup fresh orange juice (84) and 1 cup fresh pineapple slices (97).
TOTAL MEAL: 426 calories

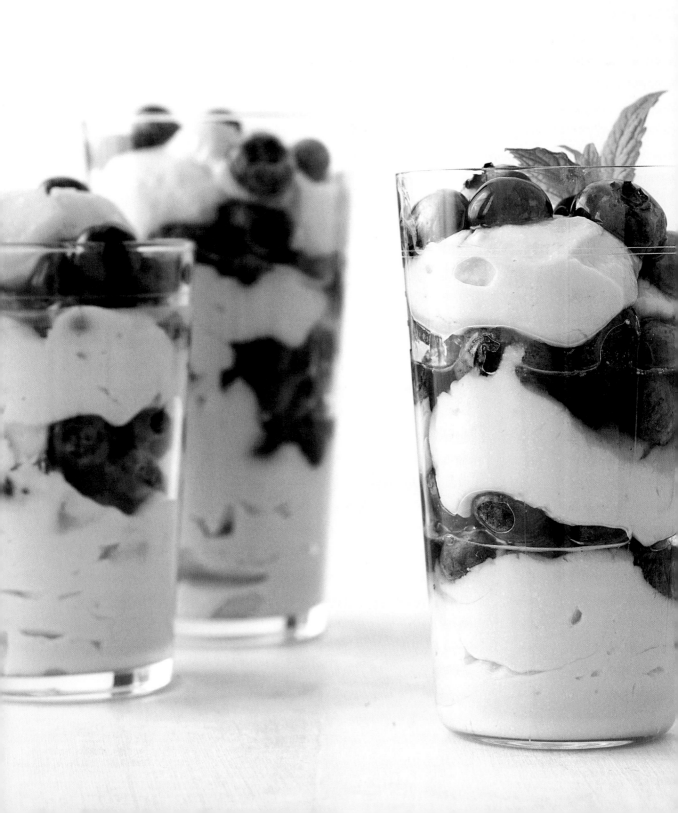

Ginger-Blueberry Parfait

■ PREP TIME: 15 MINUTES ■ TOTAL TIME: 15 MINUTES ■ MAKES 4 SERVINGS ■ MUFA: AVOCADO

When blueberry season strikes, enjoy this supereasy dessert. Blueberries provide more antioxidants than any other fresh fruit. Plus, they're grown with far fewer pesticides than many other crops.

1 cup blueberries	1 Hass avocado, peeled, pitted, and chopped
1 teaspoon grated peeled fresh ginger	1 cup part-skim ricotta cheese
4 tablespoons maple syrup, divided	4 sprigs fresh mint

1. In a small bowl, combine the blueberries, ginger, and 1 tablespoon of the maple syrup until well mixed. Let stand for 5 minutes.

2. Meanwhile, in a food processor, combine the avocado, ricotta, and the remaining 3 tablespoons maple syrup. Puree the mixture.

3. In 4 parfait glasses or dessert dishes, alternately layer the blueberry mixture with the ricotta mixture, ending with the berries. Garnish with the mint sprigs.

Nutrition per serving: 217 calories, 8 g protein, 25 g carbohydrates, 10 g total fat, 4 g saturated fat, 3 g fiber, 83 mg sodium

Make It a FLAT BELLY DIET MEAL

Serve with 2 Coconut-Almond Macaroons (page 272) (201).
TOTAL MEAL: 418 calories

Enlightened Bananas Foster

■ PREP TIME: 10 MINUTES ■ TOTAL TIME: 15 MINUTES ■ MAKES 4 SERVINGS ■ MUFA: CANOLA OIL

Ice cream itself is gluten free, but be aware of flavor combinations containing gluten. Avoid ice cream sandwiches, cones (unless they are gluten free), and flavors that include cookie dough, cheesecake, and brownie pieces.

3 tablespoons confectioners' sugar

½ teaspoon ground cinnamon, divided

4 firm-ripe bananas, sliced crosswise into 1" pieces

¼ cup canola oil

3 tablespoons honey

1 teaspoon pure vanilla extract

2 cups slow-churned reduced-fat vanilla ice cream

1. In a dish or shallow pie plate, mix together the confectioners' sugar and ¼ teaspoon of the cinnamon. Dip the cut sides of the bananas in the sugar mixture and set aside.

2. In a large nonstick skillet over medium-high heat, warm the oil. Working in batches, place the bananas, cut side down, in the skillet and cook for 2 minutes, or until browned on the bottom. Use tongs to carefully flip the pieces and cook for 1 minute. As they finish cooking, divide the banana pieces among 4 dessert dishes.

3. Remove the skillet from the heat. Carefully stir in the honey, vanilla, and the remaining ¼ teaspoon cinnamon stir until combined. Spoon the sauce over the bananas. Top each serving with ½ cup ice cream.

Nutrition per serving: 402 calories, 4 g protein, 61 g carbohydrates, 18 g total fat, 3 g saturated fat, 3 g fiber, 47 mg sodium

Make It a FLAT BELLY DIET MEAL } A single serving of this recipe counts as a Flat Belly Diet Meal without any add-ons!

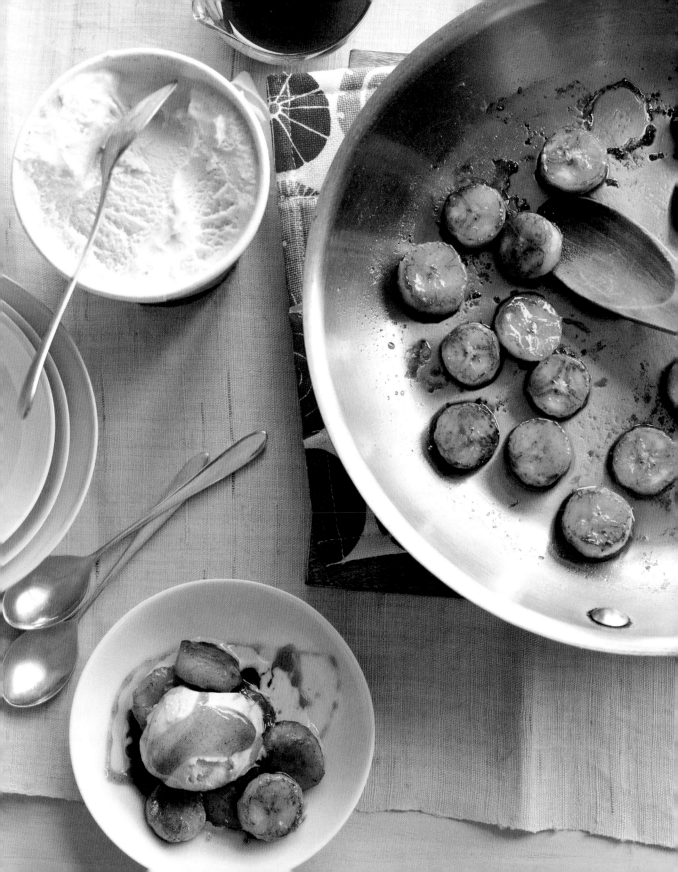

Banana, Pineapple, and Walnut Sundaes

■ PREP TIME: 10 MINUTES ■ TOTAL TIME: 15 MINUTES ■ MAKES 4 SERVINGS ■ MUFA: WALNUTS

If you have fresh pineapple on hand, you'll need about four ½-inch slices, cut into small pieces.

1 tablespoon butter

2 bananas, sliced

1 can (4 ounces) unsweetened pineapple chunks, drained well

2 tablespoons sugar

1 pint gluten-free low-fat vanilla frozen yogurt

½ cup toasted walnuts

4 maraschino cherries (optional)

1. In a medium nonstick skillet, melt the butter over medium-high heat. Add the bananas, pineapple, and sugar and cook, stirring occasionally, for 2 minutes, or until just softened and warm.

2. Scoop ½ cup of the frozen yogurt into each of 4 dessert dishes. Top with one-fourth of the fruit mixture and 2 tablespoons of the walnuts. Top each with 1 maraschino cherry, if using. Serve immediately.

Nutrition per serving: 294 calories, 6 g protein, 43 g carbohydrates, 13 g total fat, 3 g saturated fat, 3 g fiber, 85 mg sodium

Make It a FLAT BELLY DIET MEAL

Serve with 8 ounces cappuccino made with 1% milk (73).
TOTAL MEAL: 367 calories

Creamy Mango Frappé

■ PREP TIME: 10 MINUTES ■ TOTAL TIME: 10 MINUTES ■ MAKES 1 SERVING ■ MUFA: FLAXSEED OIL

For an extra boost, add 1 tablespoon gluten-free vanilla protein powder.

¼ cup part-skim ricotta cheese

1 tablespoon 1% milk

1 tablespoon flaxseed oil

1½ teaspoons honey

1 teaspoon grated orange peel

¼ cup peeled, pitted, and chopped mango

In a food processor, combine the ricotta, milk, oil, honey, and orange peel. Pulse until smooth. Pour into a tall glass. Top with the mango and serve at once.

Nutrition per serving: 279 calories, 8 g protein, 21 g carbohydrates, 19 g total fat, 5 g saturated fat, 1 g fiber, 85 mg sodium

Make It a
FLAT
BELLY
DIET
MEAL

Serve with 2 Lemon-Pine Nut Cookies (page 274) (144).
TOTAL MEAL: 423 calories

Your 14-Day
MEAL
PLAN

This meal plan is designed for a woman who wants to lose weight. Men who are trying to drop pounds should add one additional 400-calorie meal to each day.

Day 1

Broccoli and Pesto Omelet, page 85

½ gluten-free toasted English muffin spread with 1 tablespoon light butter spread

NUTRITION PER MEAL: 383 calories, 18 g protein, 25 g carbohydrates, 24 g total fat, 7 g saturated fat, 2 g fiber, 887 mg sodium

LUNCH

Cauliflower, Tomato, and Pesto Pasta Salad, page 129

Roast Beef Onion Soup, page 98

NUTRITION PER MEAL: 388 calories, 12 g protein, 40 g carbohydrates, 21 g total fat, 2.5 g saturated fat, 5 g fiber, 286 mg sodium

DINNER

Grilled Steak with Blue Cheese and Walnuts, page 198

1 cup steamed broccoli

NUTRITION PER MEAL: 397 calories, 31 g protein, 14 g carbohydrates, 26 g total fat, 7 g saturated fat, 6 g fiber, 677 mg sodium

SNACK

Roast Peaches with Pistachio-Streusel Topping, page 260

NUTRITION PER MEAL: 251 calories, 4 g protein, 26 g carbohydrates, 16 g total fat, 6 g saturated fat, 4 g fiber, 65 mg sodium

DAILY NUTRITION TOTAL: 1,419 calories, 65 g protein, 105 g carbohydrates, 87 g total fat, 22.5 g saturated fat, 17 g fiber, 1,915 mg sodium

Day 2

BREAKFAST

Orange and Dried Cherry Porridge, page 71

2 sliced plums

NUTRITION PER MEAL: 403 calories, 11 g protein, 73 g carbohydrates, 9 g total fat, 1.5 g saturated fat, 11 g fiber, 98 mg sodium

LUNCH

Creamy Gazpacho, page 105

½ Smoky Avocado BLT, page 110

1 cup cucumber slices

1 clementine

NUTRITION PER MEAL: 377 calories, 19 g protein, 41 g carbohydrates, 17 g total fat, 4 g saturated fat, 7 g fiber, 856 mg sodium

DINNER

Halibut with Chopped Olive and Potato Salad, page 172

NUTRITION PER MEAL: 350 calories, 37 g protein, 11 g carbohydrates, 18 g total fat, 2 g saturated fat, 2 g fiber, 631 mg sodium

SNACK

2 tablespoons Spice-Roasted Almonds, page 250

1 cup fresh blueberries

NUTRITION PER MEAL: 201 calories, 5 g protein, 25 g carbohydrates, 11 g total fat, 1 g saturated fat, 6 g fiber, 67 mg sodium

DAILY NUTRITION TOTAL: 1,331 calories, 71 g protein, 150 g carbohydrates, 54 g total fat, 8.5 g saturated fat, 25 g fiber, 1,651 mg sodium

Day 3

Blackberry Yogurt Parfaits, page 93

2 ounces Canadian bacon, cooked

1 hard-cooked egg

NUTRITION PER MEAL: 385 calories, 32 g protein, 31 g carbohydrates, 15 g total fat, 3.5 g saturated fat, 7 g fiber, 906 mg sodium

LUNCH

Mediterranean Salmon Salad Sandwich, page 115

Crunchy Garden Salad with Green Goddess Dressing, page 130

NUTRITION PER MEAL: 395 calories, 23 g protein, 26 g carbohydrates, 24 g total fat, 3 g saturated fat, 8 g fiber, 832 mg sodium

DINNER

Tofu, Asparagus, and Cashew Stir-Fry, page 160

½ cup brown rice

NUTRITION PER MEAL: 371 calories, 17 g protein, 40 g carbohydrates, 17 g total fat, 3 g saturated fat, 6 g fiber, 469 mg sodium

SNACK

1 gluten-free rice cake spread with 2 tablespoons unsalted natural peanut butter and topped with ¼ sliced banana

NUTRITION PER MEAL: 261 calories, 8 g protein, 21 g carbohydrates, 16 g total fat, 2 g saturated fat, 3 g fiber, 14 mg sodium

DAILY NUTRITION TOTAL: 1,411 calories, 81 g protein, 119 g carbohydrates, 73 g total fat, 11.5 g saturated fat, 23 g fiber, 2,221 mg sodium

Day 4

BREAKFAST

Chocolate-Peanut Butter Stuffed French Toast with Strawberry Sauce, page 72

NUTRITION PER MEAL: 432 calories, 14 g protein, 49 g carbohydrates, 23 g total fat, 7.5 g saturated fat, 5 g fiber, 439 mg sodium

LUNCH

Roast Chicken and Fresh Corn Salad, page 134

1 cup cubed watermelon

NUTRITION PER MEAL: 336 calories, 26 g protein, 31 g carbohydrates, 14 g total fat, 2 g saturated fat, 3 g fiber, 436 mg sodium

DINNER

Turkey Cutlets with Bacon and Avocado, page 192

1 cup roasted baby red potatoes

½ cup steamed green beans

NUTRITION PER MEAL: 377 calories, 36 g protein, 39 g carbohydrates, 9 g total fat, 1.5 g saturated fat, 7 g fiber, 357 mg sodium

SNACK

4 gluten-free multigrain crackers topped with ¼ sliced avocado, ¼ cup salsa, and 2 tablespoons shredded pepper Jack cheese

NUTRITION PER MEAL: 199 calories, 5 g protein, 17 g carbohydrates, 13 g total fat, 4 g saturated fat, 4 g fiber, 408 mg sodium

DAILY NUTRITION TOTAL: 1,344 calories, 80 g protein, 136 g carbohydrates, 59 g total fat, 15 g saturated fat, 19 g fiber, 1,640 mg sodium

Day 5

BREAKFAST

Almond Waffles with Tropical Fruit Salsa, page 76

NUTRITION PER MEAL: 418 calories, 13 g protein, 55 g carbohydrates, 19 g total fat, 2 g saturated fat, 8 g fiber, 177 mg sodium

LUNCH

Butternut Squash and Kale Soup with Pecans, page 107

Tangy Roast Beef Lettuce Wrap, page 111

NUTRITION PER MEAL: 390 calories, 20 g protein, 37 g carbohydrates, 20 g total fat, 3 g saturated fat, 8 g fiber, 675 mg sodium

DINNER

Chicken Cobbler with Cornmeal-Pepita Topping, page 186

NUTRITION PER MEAL: 406 calories, 22 g protein, 43 g carbohydrates, 17 g total fat, 3 g saturated fat, 4 g fiber, 527 mg sodium

SNACK

5 Walnut Meringues, page 275

NUTRITION PER MEAL: 143 calories, 4 g protein, 18 g carbohydrates, 7 g total fat, 1 g saturated fat, 1 g fiber, 37 mg sodium

DAILY NUTRITION TOTAL: 1,357 calories, 59 g protein, 154 g carbohydrates, 62 g total fat, 9 g saturated fat, 21 g fiber, 1,417 mg sodium

Day 6

BREAKFAST

Grab-and-Go Breakfast Cups, page 77

1 container (6 ounces) 0% plain Greek yogurt

NUTRITION PER MEAL: 361 calories, 30 g protein, 12 g carbohydrates, 21 g total fat, 5 g saturated fat, 1 g fiber, 946 mg sodium

LUNCH

Curried Cashew Chicken, page 184

½ cup cooked quinoa

NUTRITION PER MEAL: 394 calories, 29 g protein, 30 g carbohydrates, 18 g total fat, 3.5 g saturated fat, 4 g fiber, 247 mg sodium

DINNER

Smoky Pork and Sweet Potato Skillet, page 210

Zucchini Ribbons with Pine Nuts and Dill, page 215

NUTRITION PER MEAL: 435 calories, 29 g protein, 28 g carbohydrates, 25 g total fat, 3.5 g saturated fat, 7 g fiber, 426 mg sodium

SNACK

2 Lemon–Pine Nut Cookies, page 274

½ cup 1% milk

NUTRITION PER MEAL: 195 calories, 8 g protein, 18 g carbohydrates, 12 g total fat, 1.5 g saturated fat, 1 g fiber, 74 mg sodium

DAILY NUTRITION TOTAL: 1,386 calories, 96 g protein, 88 g carbohydrates, 75 g total fat, 13.5 g saturated fat, 13 g fiber, 1,693 mg sodium

Day 7

Chocolate–Peanut Butter Smoothie, page 94

1 orange

NUTRITION PER MEAL: 391 calories, 14 g protein, 45 g carbohydrates, 13 g total fat, 2.5 g saturated fat, 7 g fiber, 215 mg sodium

LUNCH

Grilled Cheese with Ham and Tomatoes, page 108

1 cup celery sticks

NUTRITION PER MEAL: 393 calories, 20 g protein, 31 g carbohydrates, 22 g total fat, 3.5 g saturated fat, 3 g fiber, 975 mg sodium

DINNER

Shrimp Jambalaya, page 180

1 cup cooked green beans

1 pear

NUTRITION PER MEAL: 411 calories, 22 g protein, 54 g carbohydrates, 13 g total fat, 1.5 g saturated fat, 13 g fiber, 721 mg sodium

SNACK

Olive Oil Cornmeal Cake, page 265

NUTRITION PER MEAL: 224 calories, 5 g protein, 22 g carbohydrates, 14 g total fat, 2 g saturated fat, 2 g fiber, 193 mg sodium

DAILY NUTRITION TOTAL: 1,419 calories, 61 g protein, 151 g carbohydrates, 62 g total fat, 9 g saturated fat, 25 g fiber, 2,105 mg sodium

Day 8

BREAKFAST

Pan-Fried Cheesy Polenta, page 79

½ cup grapes

NUTRITION PER MEAL: 419 calories, 11 g protein, 54 g carbohydrates, 20 g total fat, 4.5 g saturated fat, 3 g fiber, 384 mg sodium

LUNCH

Tuna Melt, page 114

1 apple and 2 tablespoons pistachios

NUTRITION PER MEAL: 405 calories, 23 g protein, 38 g carbohydrates, 19 g total fat, 3.5 g saturated fat, 6 g fiber, 385 mg sodium

DINNER

Shish Kebabs with Lemon-Tahini Sauce, page 206

½ cup cooked quinoa

NUTRITION PER MEAL: 404 calories, 33 g protein, 29 g carbohydrates, 18 g total fat, 3.5 g saturated fat, 6 g fiber, 96 mg sodium

SNACK

1 Peanut Butter–Chocolate Chunk Cookie, page 271

NUTRITION PER MEAL: 394 calories, 10 g protein, 36 g carbohydrates, 25 g total fat, 5 g saturated fat, 4 g fiber, 128 mg sodium

DAILY NUTRITION TOTAL: 1,621 calories, 77 g protein, 157 g carbohydrates, 81 g total fat, 16.5 g saturated fat, 18 g fiber, 992 mg sodium

Day 9

BREAKFAST

Crunchy Peanut Butter–Banana Wrap, page 92

$\frac{1}{2}$ cup fat-free milk

NUTRITION PER MEAL: 418 calories, 13 g protein, 47 g carbohydrates, 20 g total fat, 3 g saturated fat, 5 g fiber, 214 mg sodium

LUNCH

Tropical Turkey Salad, page 132

4 slices gluten-free crispbreads

NUTRITION PER MEAL: 409 calories, 32 g protein, 39 g carbohydrates, 14 g total fat, 2 g saturated fat, 6 g fiber, 521 mg sodium

DINNER

Olive-Stuffed Beef Rolls, page 200

$\frac{1}{2}$ cup cooked brown rice

NUTRITION PER MEAL: 428 calories, 40 g protein, 30 g carbohydrates, 20 g total fat, 4 g saturated fat, 3 g fiber, 531 mg sodium

SNACK

1 Cashew Brownie, page 268

NUTRITION PER MEAL: 290 calories, 5 g protein, 32 g carbohydrates, 18 g total fat, 4 g saturated fat, 3 g fiber, 127 mg sodium

DAILY NUTRITION TOTAL: 1,546 calories, 91 g protein, 147 g carbohydrates, 73 g total fat, 13 g saturated fat, 16 g fiber, 1,393 mg sodium

Day 10

BREAKFAST

Breakfast Tacos with Tomato Guacamole, page 89

1 cup reduced-sodium tomato juice

NUTRITION PER MEAL: 386 calories, 21 g protein, 44 g carbohydrates, 16 g total fat, 4 g saturated fat, 9 g fiber, 657 mg sodium

LUNCH

Pesto Chicken Caesar Salad, page 150

$\frac{1}{4}$ cup Parmesan-Pepper Croutons, page 131

NUTRITION PER MEAL: 363 calories, 27 g protein, 13 g carbohydrates, 22 g total fat, 4 g saturated fat, 3 g fiber, 327 mg sodium

DINNER

Grilled Steak with Blue Cheese and Walnuts, page 198

$\frac{1}{4}$ cup shelled, cooked edamame

NUTRITION PER MEAL: 390 calories, 31 g protein, 6 g carbohydrates, 27 g total fat, 7 g saturated fat, 3 g fiber, 615 mg sodium

SNACK

Mocha Chocolate Cake, page 263

NUTRITION PER MEAL: 402 calories, 5 g protein, 50 g carbohydrates, 23 g total fat, 6 g saturated fat, 7 g fiber, 512 mg sodium

DAILY NUTRITION TOTAL: 1,540 calories, 84 g protein, 113 g carbohydrates, 87 g total fat, 21 g saturated fat, 22 g fiber, 2,111 mg sodium

Day 11

1½ cups crispy brown rice cereal, served with 1 cup fat-free milk and topped with ½ cup blueberries and 2 tablespoons walnuts

NUTRITION PER MEAL: 407 calories, 14 g protein, 66 g carbohydrates, 12 g total fat, 1.5 g saturated fat, 6 g fiber, 110 mg sodium

LUNCH

Tuscan Tuna and White Bean Salad, page 128

1 pear

NUTRITION PER MEAL: 391 calories, 21 g protein, 45 g carbohydrates, 16 g total fat, 2.5 g saturated fat, 12 g fiber, 440 mg sodium

DINNER

Pecan-Crusted Cod, page 174

¼ pound steamed asparagus spears topped with 2 teaspoons trans-free margarine

NUTRITION PER MEAL: 387 calories, 31 g protein, 25 g carbohydrates, 19 g total fat, 2.5 g saturated fat, 5 g fiber, 614 mg sodium

SNACK

1 Dark Chocolate Fudge Pop, page 279

NUTRITION PER MEAL: 245 calories, 6 g protein, 32 g carbohydrates, 13 g total fat, 8 g saturated fat, 3 g fiber, 28 mg sodium

DAILY NUTRITION TOTAL: 1,429 calories, 72 g protein, 168 g carbohydrates, 59 g total fat, 14.5 g saturated fat, 26 g fiber, 1,191 mg sodium

Day 12

BREAKFAST

Apple and Almond Butter Sandwich, page 90

1 cup fat-free milk

NUTRITION PER MEAL: 416 calories, 15 g protein, 49 g carbohydrates, 20 g total fat, 2 g saturated fat, 2 g fiber, 456 mg sodium

LUNCH

Tzatziki Chicken Wrap, page 118

1 cup red bell pepper strips

NUTRITION PER MEAL: 352 calories, 19 g protein, 38 g carbohydrates, 14 g total fat, 1 g saturated fat, 6 g fiber, 1,158 mg sodium

DINNER

3 ounces roasted pork tenderloin

Roasted Carrots with Walnuts and Leeks, page 214

1 cup steamed broccoli topped with 2 teaspoons trans-free margarine

NUTRITION PER MEAL: 421 calories, 32 g protein, 30 g carbohydrates, 21 g total fat, 4 g saturated fat, 10 g fiber, 368 mg sodium

SNACK

1 cup Peanut Caramel Popcorn, page 247

NUTRITION PER MEAL: 251 calories, 5 g protein, 26 g carbohydrates, 15 g total fat, 5 g saturated fat, 3 g fiber, 270 mg sodium

DAILY NUTRITION TOTAL: 1,440 calories, 71 g protein, 143 g carbohydrates, 70 g total fat, 18 g saturated fat, 21 g fiber, 2,252 mg sodium

Day 13

Pomegranate-Peach Smoothie, page 94

1 slice gluten-free cinnamon-raisin bread, toasted and spread with 1 tablespoon fat-free cream cheese

NUTRITION PER MEAL: 403 calories, 7 g protein, 63 g carbohydrates, 16 g total fat, 1.5 g saturated fat, 3 g fiber, 246 mg sodium

LUNCH

3 ounces cooked sliced chicken breast

Heirloom Tomato Salad with Lemon Aioli, page 142

Almond-Saffron Rice, page 228

NUTRITION PER MEAL: 424 calories, 33 g protein, 33 g carbohydrates, 17 g total fat, 2 g saturated fat, 4 g fiber, 548 mg sodium

DINNER

Pizza Puttanesca, page 163

2 cups mixed baby greens tossed with 2 tablespoons balsamic vinaigrette

NUTRITION PER MEAL: 345 calories, 8 g protein, 32 g carbohydrates, 21 g total fat, 2.5 g saturated fat, 4 g fiber, 1,059 mg sodium

SNACK

1 Banana and Dark Chocolate Chip Cupcake, page 266

NUTRITION PER MEAL: 285 calories, 5 g protein, 35 g carbohydrates, 16 g total fat, 3 g saturated fat, 3 g fiber, 130 mg sodium

DAILY NUTRITION TOTAL: 1,457 calories, 53 g protein, 163 g carbohydrates, 70 g total fat, 9.5 g saturated fat, 14 g fiber, 1,983 mg sodium

Day 14

BREAKFAST

Cashew-Ginger Granola, page 249

6 ounces fat-free vanilla yogurt

1 cup cantaloupe cubes

NUTRITION PER MEAL: 390 calories, 15 g protein, 61 g carbohydrates, 11 g total fat, 1.5 g saturated fat, 3 g fiber, 146 mg sodium

LUNCH

Eggplant Rolls with Roasted Red Peppers and Pesto, page 162

Grilled Pear Salad with Walnuts and Pomegranate Vinaigrette, page 147

NUTRITION PER MEAL: 390 calories, 11 g protein, 34 g carbohydrates, 25 g total fat, 6 g saturated fat, 10 g fiber, 889 mg sodium

DINNER

Family-Style Spaghetti and Meatballs, page 203

1 cup cooked spinach

NUTRITION PER MEAL: 414 calories, 26 g protein, 47 g carbohydrates, 13 g total fat, 3 g saturated fat, 9 g fiber, 720 mg sodium

SNACK

2 cups Cumin-Scented Kale Chips, page 238

NUTRITION PER MEAL: 178 calories, 4 g protein, 12 g carbohydrates, 15 g total fat, 2 g saturated fat, 2 g fiber, 290 mg sodium

DAILY NUTRITION TOTAL: 1,372 calories, 56 g protein, 154 g carbohydrates, 64 g total fat, 13 g saturated fat, 24 g fiber, 2,044 mg sodium

Your MUFA SERVING CHART

FOOD	SERVING	CALORIES
Almond butter	2 Tbsp	200
Almond flour	1/4 cup	160
Almond meal	1/4 cup	160
Almond milk (unsweetened)*	1 cup	40
Almonds	2 Tbsp	109
Avocados, California (Hass)	1/4 cup	96
Avocados, Florida	1/4 cup	69
Black olive tapenade	2 Tbsp	88
Brazil nuts	2 Tbsp	110
Canola oil	1 Tbsp	124
Canola oil mayonnaise	1 Tbsp	100
Cashew butter	2 Tbsp	190
Cashews	2 Tbsp	100
Flaxseed oil (cold-pressed organic)	1 Tbsp	120
Green olive tapenade	2 Tbsp	54
Hazelnuts	2 Tbsp	110
Macadamia nuts	2 Tbsp	120
Olive oil	1 Tbsp	119
Olives (green or black)	10 large	50
Peanut butter, natural (crunchy)	2 Tbsp	188
Peanut butter, natural (smooth)	2 Tbsp	188
Peanut oil	1 Tbsp	119
Peanuts	2 Tbsp	110
Pecans	2 Tbsp	90
Pesto	1 Tbsp	80
Pine nuts	2 Tbsp	113
Pistachios	2 Tbsp	88
Pumpkin seeds	2 Tbsp	148
Safflower oil (high oleic)	1 Tbsp	120
Semisweet chocolate chips	1/4 cup	207
Sesame or soybean oil	1 Tbsp	120
Sesame seeds	2 Tbsp	91
Soybeans (edamame), shelled and boiled	1 cup	298
Sunflower oil (high oleic)	1 Tbsp	120
Sunflower seed butter	2 Tbsp	190
Sunflower seeds	2 Tbsp	90
Tahini (sesame seed paste)	2 Tbsp	178
Walnut oil	1 Tbsp	120
Walnuts	2 Tbsp	82

*The brand we recommend, Almond Breeze, is gluten free.

Your GLUTEN-FREE SUBSTITUTIONS LIST

On the following pages, you'll find substitutions for flour and grains. If you're allergic to milk, eggs, or other ingredients, you'll find substitutions for them, too.

Flour

Replacement Flours and Starches

GRAIN FLOURS AND STARCHES	LEGUME FLOURS	SEED FLOURS	TUBER FLOURS AND STARCHES	NUT FLOURS
Rice	Soy	Flaxseed	Potato	Chestnut
Corn	Chickpea	Buckwheat	Tapioca	Almond
Sorghum	Fava bean	Amaranth	Arrowroot	Walnut
Millet		Quinoa	Sweet potato	Hazelnut

Per cup: When you substitute gluten-free flour for all-purpose flour, use 2 tablespoons less flour per cup. So, when a recipe calls for 1 cup of all-purpose flour, substitute ⅞ cup of a gluten-free flour.

Per tablespoon: For 1 tablespoon of wheat flour, substitute one of these:

- 1½ teaspoons cornstarch
- 1½ teaspoons potato starch
- 1½ teaspoons arrowroot starch
- 1½ teaspoons rice flour
- 2 teaspoons quick-cooking tapioca

For 1 cup of wheat flour, substitute one of these:

- ¾ cup plain cornmeal, coarse
- 1 cup plain cornmeal, fine
- ⅝ cup potato flour
- ¾ cup rice flour

All-Purpose Gluten-Free Flour Blend

You can use this blend for gluten-free breads, muffins, cookies, and more.

- ½ cup rice flour
- ¼ cup tapioca starch/flour
- ¼ cup cornstarch or potato starch

Combine all of the ingredients and store in a covered container in the refrigerator until used. You can double or triple this recipe to make as much as you need.

Milk

Replace 1 cup of cow's milk with an equal amount of:

- Water
- Soy milk (plain)
- Rice milk
- Goat's milk, if tolerated
- Hemp milk

Eggs

Replace 1 large egg with one of the following:

- 3 tablespoons unsweetened applesauce (or other fruit puree) + 1 teaspoon baking powder
- 1 tablespoon flax meal, chia seed, or salba seed + 3 tablespoons hot water (Let stand, stirring occasionally, about 10 minutes or until thick. Use without straining.)
- Egg Replacer, according to package directions
- 4 tablespoons pureed silken tofu + 1 teaspoon baking powder

Replacing more than 2 eggs will change the integrity of a recipe. For recipes that call for a lot of eggs, like a quiche, use pureed silken tofu. Because egg substitutions add moisture, you may have to increase baking times slightly.

Yogurt

Replace 1 cup of yogurt with an equal amount of:

- Soy or coconut yogurt
- Soy sour cream
- Unsweetened applesauce
- Fruit puree

Butter

Replace 8 tablespoons (1 stick) of butter with an equal amount of:

- Vegetable or olive oil
- Fleischmann's unsalted margarine
- Earth Balance Natural Buttery Spread (nondairy)
- Spectrum Organic Shortening

resources

Use this section to find the best brands, organizations, and Web sites to locate gluten-free meals and ingredients, as well as to learn more about celiac disease and non-celiac gluten sensitivity.

IN YOUR GROCERY STORE

Preparing the hearty, delicious gluten-free meals in this cookbook is easy when you know where to look for the best ingredients. Below we have included a list of gluten-free brands that should be easy to find in your local supermarket—but be sure to ask your grocer to stock up if they don't already carry them.

GLUTEN-FREE BRANDS

Andrea's Gluten Free
759 Spirit of St. Louis Blvd.
Chesterfield, MO 63005
636-536-9953
andreasglutenfree.com

Applegate Farms
750 Rt. 202 South, Suite 300
Bridgewater, NJ 08807-5530
866-587-5858
applegate.com

Authentic Foods
1850 W. 169th Street, Suite B
Gardena, CA 90247
800-806-4737
authenticfoods.com

Bob's Red Mill
13521 SE Pheasant Ct.
Milwaukie, OR 97222
503-654-3215
bobsredmill.com/gluten-free/

Canyon Bakehouse
canyonbakehouse.com

Crunchmaster
800-896-2396
crunchmaster.com

Enjoy Life Foods
3810 River Road
Schiller Park, IL 60176
847-260-0300
enjoylifefoods.com

Glutino
115 West Century Road,
    Suite 260
Paramus, NJ 07652
201-421-3970
glutino.com

Katz Gluten Free
51 Forest Road, Suite 316 #58
Monroe, NY 10950
845-782-5307
katzglutenfree.com

Lundberg Family Farms
5311 Midway
P.O. Box 369
Richvale, CA 95974
530-538-3500
lundberg.com

**Maplegrove Gluten Free
    Foods, Inc.**
13112 Santa Ana Ave.
Fontana, CA 92337
909-823-8230
maplegrovefoods.com

Namaste Foods, LLC
P.O. Box 3133
Coeur d'Alene, ID 83816
866-258-9493
namastefoods.com

Rudi's Gluten-Free Bakery
3300 Walnut St., Unit C
Boulder, CO 80301
303-447-0495
rudisglutenfree.com

Schär
1050 Wall Street West,
    Suite 370
Lyndhurst, NJ 07071
schar.com/us/

Udi's Gluten Free
12000 E. 47th Avenue,
    Suite 400
Denver, CO 80239
201-421-3970
udisglutenfree.com/

Mary's Gone Crackers
P.O. Box 965
Gridley, CA 95948
888-258-1250
marysgonecrackers.com

ONLINE GROCERIES

Gluten-Free Mall
celiac.com/glutenfreemall

**Gluten-Free Trading
    Company**
gluten-free.net

Gluten Solutions
glutensolutions.com

IN YOUR NEIGHBORHOOD

When you're not in the mood to cook, these are just a few of the many online resources available to help you find healthy, local gluten-free dining options.

Celiac Restaurant Guide
celiacrestaurantguide.com

Find Me Gluten Free
findmeglutenfree.com

G-Free Foodie
gfreefoodie.com

Gluten Free Registry
glutenfreeregistry.com

The Gluten-Free Restaurant Awareness Program
glutenfreerestaurants.org

ORGANIZATIONS AND RESEARCH CENTERS

You can contact these organizations for more information on celiac disease, gluten insensitivity, and living a gluten-free lifestyle.

American Celiac Disease Alliance (ACDA)
2504 Duxbury Place
Alexandria, VA 22308
703-622-3331
americanceliac.org

Food Allergy Research & Education (FARE)
7925 Jones Branch Drive, Suite 1100
McLean, VA 22102
800-929-4040
foodallergy.org

Gluten Intolerance Group
31214 124th Avenue SE
Auburn, WA 98092-3667
253-833-6655
gluten.net

National Foundation for Celiac Awareness (NFCA)
P.O. Box 544
Ambler, PA 19002-0544
215-325-1306
celiaccentral.org

National Institutes of Health (NIH)
Celiac Disease Awareness Campaign
c/o National Digestive Diseases
Information Clearinghouse
2 Information Way
Bethesda, MD 20892-3570
800-891-5389
celiac.nih.gov

index

Underscored page references indicate sidebars and tables. **Boldface** references indicate photographs.

conversion chart

These equivalents have been slightly rounded to make measuring easier.

VOLUME MEASUREMENTS			WEIGHT MEASUREMENTS		LENGTH MEASUREMENTS	
U.S.	IMPERIAL	METRIC	U.S.	METRIC	U.S.	METRIC
¼ tsp	–	1 ml	1 oz	30 g	¼"	0.6 cm
½ tsp	–	2 ml	2 oz	60 g	½"	1.25 cm
1 tsp	–	5 ml	4 oz (¼ lb)	115 g	1"	2.5 cm
1 Tbsp	–	15 ml	5 oz (⅓ lb)	145 g	2"	5 cm
2 Tbsp (1 oz)	1 fl oz	30 ml	6 oz	170 g	4"	11 cm
¼ cup (2 oz)	2 fl oz	60 ml	7 oz	200 g	6"	15 cm
⅓ cup (3 oz)	3 fl oz	80 ml	8 oz (½ lb)	230 g	8"	20 cm
½ cup (4 oz)	4 fl oz	120 ml	10 oz	285 g	10"	25 cm
⅔ cup (5 oz)	5 fl oz	160 ml	12 oz (¾ lb)	340 g	12" (1')	30 cm
¾ cup (6 oz)	6 fl oz	180 ml	14 oz	400 g		
1 cup (8 oz)	8 fl oz	240 ml	16 oz (1 lb)	455 g		
			2.2 lb	1 kg		

PAN SIZES		TEMPERATURES		
U.S.	METRIC	FAHRENHEIT	CENTIGRADE	GAS
8" cake pan	20 × 4 cm sandwich or cake tin	140°	60°	–
9" cake pan	23 × 3.5 cm sandwich or cake tin	160°	70°	–
11" × 7" baking pan	28 × 18 cm baking tin	180°	80°	–
13" × 9" baking pan	32.5 × 23 cm baking tin	225°	105°	¼
15" × 10" baking pan	38 × 25.5 cm baking tin	250°	120°	½
	(Swiss roll tin)	275°	135°	1
1½ qt baking dish	1.5 liter baking dish	300°	150°	2
2 qt baking dish	2 liter baking dish	325°	160°	3
2 qt rectangular baking dish	30 × 19 cm baking dish	350°	180°	4
9" pie plate	22 × 4 or 23 × 4 cm pie plate	375°	190°	5
7" or 8" springform pan	18 or 20 cm springform or	400°	200°	6
	loose-bottom cake tin	425°	220°	7
9" × 5" loaf pan	23 × 13 cm or 2 lb narrow	450°	230°	8
	loaf tin or pâté tin	475°	245°	9
		500°	260°	–